P9-EDN-772

The Redux™ Revolution

The Redux™ Revolution

Sheldon Levine, M.D.

William Morrow and Company, Inc.

New York

The ideas, procedures, and suggestions contained in this book are not intended to substitute for the help and services of a trained professional. All matters regarding your health require medical consultation and supervision, and following any of the advice and procedures in this book should be done in conjunction with the services of a qualified health professional.

The names and identifying characteristics of the individuals referred to in anecdotes in this book have been changed to protect the identity of the individuals concerned.

Copyright © 1996 by Sheldon Levine, M.D.

Redux™ is a trademark of ORSEM (SERVIER). This work was neither written nor published with the approval or sponsorship of Orsem (Servier), or of any other entity.

All rights reserved. No part of this book may be reproduced or utilized in any form or by any means, electronic or mechanical, including photo-copying, recording, or by any information storage or retrieval system, without permission in writing from the Publisher. Inquiries should be addressed to Permissions Department, William Morrow and Company, Inc., 1350 Avenue of the Americas, New York, N.Y. 10019.

It is the policy of William Morrow and Company, Inc., and its imprints and affiliates, recognizing the importance of preserving what has been written, to print the books we publish on acid-free paper, and we exert our best efforts to that end.

Library of Congress Cataloging-in-Publication Data

Levine, Sheldon.
The Redux™ revolution / Sheldon Levine.
p.   cm.
Includes bibliographical references and index.
ISBN 0-688-15153-1
1. Dexfenfluramine.   2. Obesity—Chemotherapy.   3. Weight loss.
I. title.
RC628.L39   1996
616.3'98061—dc20   96-26000
                                                                CIP

Printed in the United States of America

First Edition

1 2 3 4 5 6 7 8 9 10

BOOK DESIGN BY SUSAN HOOD

—To Janette, my wife:
A humble thank-you for all your sacrifices. Your intelligence and beauty provide perfect nourishment for body and soul.

—To my children, Alison and David:
Two total loves and the gatekeepers of the next millennium.

—To my parents and teachers, Sol and Bella:
A lifetime of unwavering gratitude for sharing your wisdom, honesty, and spirituality. It is an honor to be your son.

Acknowledgments

A book is much more than a compilation of ideas on pages: It is a collaboration of people. I am very grateful to everyone who played a part in *The Redux™ Revolution*. Two special people who were nurturing and supportive from the very beginning are Richard and Ilana Rindner, Ph.D., my in-laws. Their son, Marc, provided invaluable legal advice.

A warm thank-you to all those at William Morrow & Company involved in this project. Senior editor Toni Sciarra deserves a great deal of credit and appreciation. Toni has orchestrated and guided *The Redux™ Revolution* from its inception. It was her ability to grasp new concepts and crystallize in words the most complex scientific information and her grace while working within very limited time constraints that enabled *The Redux™ Revolution* to come to fruition. Thank you, Toni. I would also like to extend thanks to Toni's assistant, Katharine Cluverius, who helped steer the book along

Acknowledgments

each step of the way, and to Alexia Dorszynski for her invaluable assistance.

Thank you to a very special group of friends who gave time from their busy lives to help, each in his or her own way: Andrew D.P.M. and Laurie Rubin; Luigi and Anna Bellotti; Larry and Francine Goldberg, Esq.; Hal and Marti Rifkin; and the DiScala family: Reno DiScala, M.D.; Susan, Nicholas, and Alexander; and Bart and Ellen Gorrin.

To a unique individual who gave encouragement all the way: friend, chef, adventurer, and mentor Lawrence Wilkinson, M.D.

Thanks to those who helped shape my medical thinking:

From Mt. Carmel Mercy Hospital in Detroit: Leonard Alexander, M.D.; Frank Check, M.D.; Robert Schaffer, M.D.; David Axelrod, M.D.; Harvey Organek, M.D.; Leslie Pean, M.D.; Mahmed Sipahi, M.D.; Prince Eubanks, M.D.; Blaine Tacia, M.D.; José Hernandez, M.D.; K. Thavarajah, M.D.; P. Babhu, M.D.; and Celeste Wojcak, R.N.

From the Albert Einstein College of Medicine, Department of Pediatric Allergy and Immunology: Arye Rubinstein, M.D.; Marc Sicklick, M.D.; Larry Bernstein, M.D.; Brian Novick, M.D.; Harris Goldstein, M.D.; Andrew Wisnia, M.D.; Theresa Calvelli, Ph.D.; David Rosenstreich, M.D.; and Joseph Grizzanti, D.O.

I also want to thank Jeffery Weissberg, M.D.; Joseph Sozio, M.D.; Ken Goldman, M.D.; Vincent Andreano, M.D.; Stan Bennett; Christine Gileno; Linda G'Froehrer; Crestina Adolfini, R.N.; Jo Mary Pescatore; Brother Gerald Warren; Joan McPhillips; Shirley Sullivan; Mike Lally; Fern Segal; and Ali Yazadian.

Thank you to all the folks at Mahwah Valley Radiology: Michael D. Green, M.D.; Sue Worth; Andrew Kolar; Arthur Provost; and Lisa Schaper.

Acknowledgments

A special thanks to my brother-in-law, Uri Ascher, my niece, Donna Ascher, and my nephew, Amir Ascher, and to Antonio Settanni and Donato (Tzi-Tzi).

I am extremely grateful to Claudia Allocco, M.L.S., the director of the medical library at the Valley Hospital in Ridgewood, New Jersey, for her help in researching pertinent medical literature.

No project moves without the knowing consent of my office manager, Betty Del Pozzo. Thanks also to her daughter, Jeanine Del Pozzo, a talented writer, who met deadlines square-on and prepared the original manuscript. She received her first and last lesson in reading a doctor's handwriting. Good job, Jeanine.

A very special tribute goes to all the wonderful patients I have met through the years, each with a fascinating life history. Without you, this book would not have been possible. Your continuing weight-loss success is an inspiration to us all.

And finally, to a sister who has stood by me since we were in diapers. Thank you, Arlene, you are one of a kind.

Contents

A Note to My Patients and to Readers of This Book

Weight loss is really about not accepting the physical limits imposed both from within and from nature herself. The ability to voluntarily change one's form seems to be a treasure that can only be enjoyed by us humans. It is a noble endeavor. This book is a tribute to those patients who had the vision and courage to opt for change. They were the vanguard of the revolution. Now it's your turn.

The Redux™ Revolution

Chapter 1

What Is the
Redux Revolution?

If you're like many overweight people, you've been trying to lose weight for years. You've tried the diets—high-carbohydrate, low protein; high protein, low carbohydrate; low-fat; all-fruit; all-rice. You've been through the revolving door at the weight-loss centers and you've drunk enough slimming shakes to float an ocean liner. You've tried walking, running, and "Sweatin' to the Oldies." You may have lost some weight on one or more of these plans, but sooner or later, your appetite rebounds, and those pounds you've lost come right back—and maybe even some more on top of them. You avoid wearing shorts or a bathing suit, and if you don't already have high blood pressure or diabetes or heart disease, you worry about developing one or more of these problems associated with being overweight.

Or maybe it's simply that you've put on twenty pounds since you graduated from high school or college and try as you might, you just can't budge them. And you're concerned about the reports that seem to indicate that even putting on that modest amount of weight may put you at greater risk for cardiovascular disease.

Well, now there's finally good news on the weight-loss front. In fact, we are now in the midst of a true weight-loss revolution. Soon you will be a full-fledged, card-carrying member! I call this revolution the Redux* Revolution, because it involves Redux™ (dexfenfluramine), the new prescription weight-loss medication approved by the FDA in April 1996. But the Redux Revolution isn't just about you and your doctor deciding whether or not this potent appetite suppressant is right for you. The Redux Revolution also encompasses changing the way you've thought about diet and exercise your whole life and learning the difference between "willpower" (which doesn't work) and "discipline" (which does). The Redux Revolution is about rethinking your notions of healthy weight and body size and using the very latest biochemical tools available to help you ensure that the weight you've lost stays off for good.

As we'll see in the chapters ahead, the Redux Revolution is the happy result of the convergence of two major lines of medical research—a veritable explosion of scientific information that will challenge your own perceptions of why you are overweight and what you can do about it. The beating of the drums began in 1994, with the discovery of the gene that controls obesity, and its associated hormone, leptin. The drumbeats got louder when researchers began to piece together the puzzle of the mysterious "Syndrome X" and insulin resistance. And then when research in the area of

---

*Redux™ is a trademark of ORSEM (SERVIER). This work was neither written nor published with the approval or sponsorship of Orsem (Servier), or of any other entity.

depression yielded the fascinating information that certain neurotransmitters in the brain actually seem to control appetite, the stage was set for the FDA's approval of Redux, the small white capsule that very well may change the landscape of weight loss in America.

We'll discuss the science in detail in the coming chapters, but the driving force behind the Redux Revolution is simple: Contrary to what most people have believed for years, obesity is not the product of laziness or lack of character. Rather, it is in large part the product of genetics. And since that is the case, the idea that treatment for obesity revolves exclusively around diet and exercise is archaic. In fact, I would say that telling an overweight person "If only you ate less, you would be thin" is about as helpful as telling a wheelchair-bound person "If only you could walk, you would not be confined to a wheelchair."

The message of hope that Redux brings is based on a radical shift in thinking on the part of the medical community. At an ever-quickening pace, sophisticated biochemical research is providing undeniable evidence that *overweight people are special! Their bodies are different from those of thin and normal-weight people! And they don't react the way other people do to diet and exercise!* (But I'll bet you already knew that.)

Research shows that most overweight people have a form of biochemical imbalance. Internally, the body of an overweight person actually functions differently from that of a thin person. The differences range from the makeup of the brain to the function of the stomach, hormones, and fat cells. It is unfair and unrealistic to expect that people with different body types and body chemistries will respond the same way to conventional weight-loss diet and exercise plans.

This new understanding is essential to understanding the Redux Revolution. It explains, for the first time, why traditional diet and exercise programs don't help overweight people lose weight. Diet and exercise, by themselves, are much more conducive to keeping thin people thin. The biochemical imbalance also offers explanations for questions that have left so many overweight people discouraged and confused, such as why many overweight people actually gain weight after dieting, why some overweight people do not actually eat a great deal but remain heavy, and why still others are literally addicted to food and eat constantly.

In light of the cutting-edge research on the obesity gene, the usual doctor's prescription of "eat less and exercise more" is no longer a viable treatment for overweight people. As we'll see, the pace of scientific research has quickened, and we must all keep up. This is especially true in the field of medicine, which, incidentally, is full of obese professionals. When you see obese doctors, nurses, or psychologists, you have to ask whether these people are as up-to-date on recent developments in weight loss as they might be. Are they giving you a health message based on the understandings of yesterday, rather than of today?

What we are now learning is that the solution to the weight-loss problem lies within our bodies. *The Redux™ Revolution* will enable you to learn, listen to, and heed the "Body Rules" (explained in Chapter 5). After reading this book, you will have a new respect for your body. You will stop struggling with it, stop hating it, and instead become its ally. And this is important. After all, you can't abandon your body. You need the "old bod" to get to the new one!

In my case, the "old bod" weighed 248 pounds (though I was only 6'2"), was apple-shaped, and was unhealthy. Daily 1½-hour workouts with weights did little to help me lose fat, nor did my occasional forays into the realm of high-protein/low-fat diets. As I'll tell you in greater detail in Chapter 6, three years ago, quite by chance, I stopped fighting my body and I lost 60 pounds. My waist went from 40 inches to a much slimmer and healthier 31 inches. My own weight-loss experience provided the inspiration to devote my medical practice to helping people lose weight. The weight-loss plan contained in *The Redux™ Revolution* is based on the latest findings from the front lines of medical research, my own personal weight-loss experience, and my clinical experience with over 2,000 patients. You can be the next success story!

This Is Not a Diet Book

If you haven't peeked in the back of the book yet, do so now. You will notice there are no recipes, no menus, no portion-control lists, and no exercise diagrams. And for a simple reason: These are all weight-loss tools developed in response to knowledge gained from the 1950s to the 1970s, when restrictive diets and exercise were considered to be the only way to lose weight. But the information in this book is based on knowledge gained in the last decade—some in the last twelve months—and it presents a revolution of new ideas! *The Redux™ Revolution* isn't a diet book, it is a weight-loss book. The entire book is based on a plan to lose fat—not muscle or water—and lose it for good. You certainly cannot be expected to use a cutting-edge weight-controlling medication like Redux (or its cousin, a combination of medications called phen/fen) with outmoded diets and exercise plans. This book will not only introduce you to Redux and show you how to use it and phen/fen to your best advantage, it will provide a precise prescription for permanent weight-loss.

This weight-loss revolution comes just in time. The mood of the people is ugly. I sense a deep frustration within patients, a lack of self-confidence in their ability to lose weight. Almost daily in my work with overweight patients, I hear these painful statements repeatedly: "When I was younger it was so much easier," "I've tried almost everything," "Diet and exercise are too hard—they don't work for me," "I have yo-yoed so many times, I just can't do it anymore." Many people have suffered so many weight-loss victories and defeats that they deserve to be generals! *The Redux™ Revolution* urges you to step on that battlefield to fight your fat nemesis one more time—the last time. But this time you'll have the advantage: You'll be armed with Redux and the latest weight-loss information. So armed, you'll be able to retire from the weight-loss wars, once and for all.

I don't use the term "war" lightly. Sure, it's wonderful to lose weight and look good in every piece of clothing you own, but weight loss is important for life-and-death reasons as well. Each year in the United States there are 300,000 obesity-related deaths from such diseases as high blood pressure, diabetes, and heart disease—diseases that can often be prevented, controlled, and even cured with quite modest weight loss. Researchers have even given a new name to this cluster of life-threatening clinical signs and symptoms—Syndrome X. Syndrome X identifies a genetic predisposition to cardiovascular disease that affects some 30 million Americans. However, I don't want to frighten you into losing weight. Fright has proved to be a poor motivation for weight loss, and this book is not about fear. This book is about looking better and being healthier—which *is* possible, no matter how many times you've tried before.

A Boomer's Story

When we look at the overwhelming statistics—an estimated 60 million Americans are classified as obese today, a huge jump just in the last 40 years—we can't help but ask: How did we get to this point? What has happened within our culture that has led to such widespread problems with weight? The answer is found where most are: in history.

Let's go back in time to August 1945. World War II had just ended. From the bombed-out cities of Europe and the jungles of Malaysia, millions of GIs returned to the States. Their drive to procreate was strong, and procreate they did! They created the single largest population spurt in our history: the Baby Boomers. These children came into the world at a time of unprecedented economic growth in America. Confidence in the government was high, and American industry was king. Television was becoming our nocturnal pastime. (What *did* we do at night before it was invented?) Weaned on Uncle Miltie, Burns and Allen, and *Howdy Doody*, the Boomers graduated to *Annie Oakley, Zorro,* and *Dragnet*. They played with Mr. Machine, Candyland, and a cute new doll called Barbie. And they ate, along with their parents. New foods and food technology seemed to spring up overnight. Corn Flakes, Wheat Chex, and the humble bowl of oatmeal were swept away in a sea of sugar-filled breakfast cereals. Hundreds of companies arose to challenge the supremacy of Hershey's chocolate. We were awash in doughnuts, Scooter Pies, and the products of thousands of local ice cream factories, and the first 100 hamburgers were sold at a small roadside take-out joint (any guesses what its name was?).

In this new milieu of endlessly available, easy-to-find, easy-to-eat food, which continues to the present day, the Boomers and their families had 24-hour access to fat-laden foods. No amount of exercise could keep up with this onslaught of calories, and none ever will! Though there had always been some overweight people, now extra weight was accumulating for many more people, and they began flocking to the newly created diet centers for help in "watching their weight." These centers were the "only game in town," and to their credit, they pioneered group weight-loss therapy and were the first to recognize the importance of psychological counseling as a weight-loss tool. Initial success stories fueled the birth of the weight-loss industry, which today is a $50-billion-a-year giant. However, consumers' spirits were tempered when it was noted that 95 to 98 of every 100 people who lost weight at these centers eventually regained it. That's a 2% to 5% success rate, the same success rate that such centers have today! The diet gurus forgot to tell their patrons that they didn't have a solution for the "maintenance" problem. Almost everyone who loses weight on one of these plans eventually gains it back—and then some! To put the diet industry's 2% success rate in medical perspective, some "terminal" cancers have a spontaneous remission rate of 2%. That means that out of every 100 patients who contract these illnesses, perhaps two will get better by themselves. In other words, your chances of "beating" obesity at a commercial weight-loss center or by following a standard diet yourself are the same as your chances of overcoming "terminal" cancer with no medical treatment!

In fairness to the commercial weight-loss industry, we must admit that early practitioners simply didn't have knowledge of biochemical imbalances, obesity genes, or Redux and were relying on the diet plans of 40 years ago. And we must also acknowledge that being overweight is a complex issue, with more than one cause. For instance, though some 60 million Americans are overweight, some 160 million others are not—even though everyone has access to the same fat- and carbohydrate-laden diet. And though the genetic links we've seen with the discovery of the obesity gene are exciting, they don't offer the complete answer, either, because they cannot account for all cases of obesity. For example, why are poor women six times more likely to be overweight than affluent women? Is depression a factor in obesity? If so, then why are there many people who are depressed, yet remain thin?

These are important questions, and researchers are still seeking answers. For now, let's move on and see what has become of all those postwar love children and their parents.

In My "Weighting" Room

Fast forward to August 1996. That small hamburger restaurant I mentioned earlier has grown tremendously and has sold billions of hamburgers worldwide. And the American population keeps eating those Scooter Pies and other, newer desserts, which helps account for the fact that so many Boomers are overweight. Since there is a genetic link to obesity, the potential for overweight was always there, but the constant presence of so much high-fat food has led to much more expression of the obesity gene—that is, to much more obesity—in many more people.

The waiting room outside my office is filled with pear- and apple-shaped men and women, ranging from age 30 to 50. There are more women than men, and the weights tend to range between 150 and 320 pounds. That huge postwar baby-making epoch has now given rise to the largest population of the obese: the Boomers. Their parents are here, too.

Appallingly, so are their children. In fact, these children are getting heavier at rates greater than their parents. The recent discovery of the obesity gene helps explain this familial link. If both parents are overweight, there is an 80% chance that their offspring will be obese as well. (If one parent is over-weight, the chance of having overweight children slips to 40%. If neither parent is overweight, the chance is only 10%.) Obesity is, in large part, a genetic biochemical disorder. My waiting room is a living laboratory of proof. As we shall see, even our appetites have some genetic basis.

Mentally, I divide my overweight patients into two groups: "Pencils"—those who probably don't have an overly domi-neering obesity gene—and "Zeppelins"—those who do. Pencils can gain a good deal of weight, but they haven't been overweight all their lives and their weight tends to cluster around their middles. Zeppelins, on the other hand, are likely to be very heavy all over—their arms and legs, as well as their bellies and hips—and to have been heavy since childhood. Another way to look at the two groups of patients is to di-vide them into "hypertrophic" and "hyperplastic" people. Hyperplastic people actually have more fat cells than av-erage, and were born this way. In addition, their fat cells can grow in number and size and are distributed around their entire bodies. They are the most difficult to treat, yet Re-dux holds promise for them, too. Hypertrophic people, by contrast, have less marked obesity. They tend to have the usual "middle-aged spread"—a "beer belly" or "thunder thighs"—which they acquire as adults. Though these patients are overweight, they do not have an increase in the number of fat cells in their body, only in the size of those fat cells. This makes it easier for them to lose weight than it is for hyperplastic people. Do you know which type you are?

Knowing which category you fall into can have a profound

effect on your weight loss and health. We will explore this in detail in Chapter 2. There you will also learn what your weight-loss prognosis is.

A Question of Terminology: "Are You Obese?"

Though most of us care very much about how we look, it's important to realize that having extra fat on your body is not just a cosmetic "padding" problem. Fat is not an inert substance. It is very much alive and can create biochemical havoc in our bodies when it is out of control. And if you are overweight, your fat is out of control.

My patients come to me for treatment not just because they are overweight; they do so because they suffer from the health hazards of obesity, or are afraid, with reason, that they soon will. They have high blood pressure and take a myriad of side-effect-loaded medications to control it. They have diabetes and its much-feared complications. Some have gout. Some have arthritis. Some have had heart attacks. And many of these people are only in their 30s, 40s, and 50s! All of these ailments can be prevented, controlled, and often cured with weight loss. The Redux Revolution is here to help accomplish all of these things.

Thus far, we've been using the term "obese." Now, you may not consider yourself obese at all. Perhaps you are only "slightly heavy" or "carrying a few extra pounds." You may be stunned to learn that being merely 20% over the ideal body weight—that is, for example, weighing 168 pounds when your ideal weight is 140, or 228 pounds when your ideal weight is 190—not only defines you as obese, but also puts you at an increased risk for disease!

The word "obesity" comes from the Latin *ab* ("above")

11

and *edere* ("to eat"). It literally means "overeating," but because overeating isn't the only factor involved in obesity, the literal meaning is inadequate. For instance, when we take an in-depth view of the obesity gene later in this book, we will discover that this gene is also present in people who are only moderately overweight or even thin. In fact, since in all likelihood we'll soon find out that the "obesity" gene controls more than overweight, it's probably a poorly chosen and even somewhat misleading term for the gene. However, it is important, for the free exchange of scientific information, that we use a common language, so we're stuck with the name for the present. For the sake of simplicity, we'll use the word "obesity" interchangeably with "overweight" and the term "obesity gene" instead of "the gene that has something important to do with obesity."

How Much Should I Weigh?

A question I am frequently asked by my patients is "How much should I weigh?" Well, thanks to your tax dollars, a new answer recently arrived.

Until relatively recently, the ideal-weight-range tables that every dieter and most physicians relied on were essentially the tables developed by the insurance companies. Thus, the notion of how much a person should weigh was based on a premise that the insurance companies figured out decades ago, which is just now seeping into our popular consciousness: The more you weigh, the shorter your life span. A recent longevity and obesity study, performed on a large population of nurses, bears out this concept. Being as little as 22 pounds over your high school weight puts you at risk for early mortality.

The following graph showing Optimum Body Weight Ranges for Men and Women is from the 1995 Report of the Dietary Guidelines Advisory Committee on the Dietary Guidelines for Americans.

BMI RISK CHART

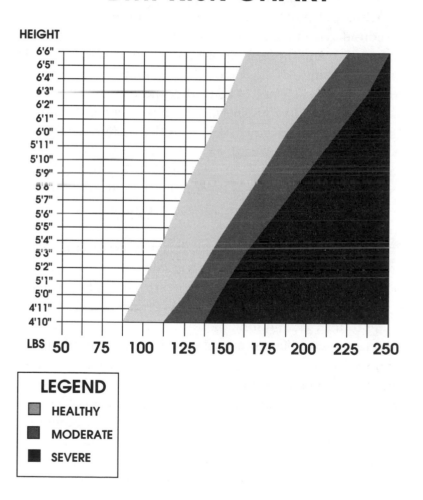

While I know that there are difficulties with using one standard chart for many individuals, the ranges shown on this chart are useful in measuring levels of *health risk*, rather than just weight. Based on these criteria—what are the health risks at different weights?—60 million Americans are obese. The average American adult woman is 5'4" tall and weighs 144 pounds; the healthy weight range for women of that height is 112 to 144 pounds. A woman of the same height would be considered obese if she weighed 173 pounds. A healthy American man who is 5'10" tall should weigh between 135 and 173 pounds. If he weighs 204 pounds or more, he is considered obese. I doubt that either the woman or the man in the examples I've given would consider herself or himself obese. I doubt that they would consider themselves actively at risk for cardiovascular disease. But they are! This point is germane to the message of *The Redux™ Revolution*. If you weigh 20% or more above the healthy body weight for your height in the chart, you must lose weight if you want to consider yourself *healthy*.

Aesthetics—how attractive we feel our bodies are—is another issue. We all want to look good, but many of us have distorted body images, whether in the direction of heaviness or thinness. This is probably due to years of watching TV shows, going to movies, and looking at magazines depicting people with thin bodies. This distorted self-image can contribute not only to obesity, but also to a disease at the other extreme—anorexia, a condition in which some of the patients weigh less than 85 pounds and still believe they are heavy.

But distortion is most common in the other direction. Let's consider one of my patients, E.M., a 35-year-old public relations director for a noted dance company, who came into my office in tears the other day. She is 5'3" and weighs 245 pounds. She told me that she had never realized how heavy she was until the previous day, when the company held an open rehearsal and she spent the entire day surrounded by very beautiful, very thin dancers. At this point, I realized something very important: Although I had been treating E.M. for two months, I had missed a key point in her treatment. Though I thought we were in agreement about where we were starting from, she was in deep denial about her weight. In her mind, she was "only a little bit heavy" and had to lose "only a few pounds." We decided that the best course of action would be for her to see a psychologist; when she had successfully dealt with her sense of her body, she could then pursue weight loss.

I see another common distortion when I ask heavy women, at serious risk for cardiovascular disease, to describe their husbands. They invariably describe them as either "slightly heavy" or "thin." When I finally meet these men, I am always surprised to see how heavy they actually are. The women's responses are not so much falsehoods as differences in perception, distortion of body images, and fantasy. We often see others as thinner or heavier based on our own distorted body perception. This inability to see oneself undistorted in the present often interferes with weight loss in the future.

Health and Weight

How do I answer patients when they ask me what they should weigh? One of the problems with the government Optimum Body Weight Ranges chart is that it does not take age into consideration.

As we age, we tend to deposit fat. The same is true for most mammals. This is considered to be a normal process and has nothing to do with eating habits or genetics—that is, it's true of both healthy, normal-weight people and the obese. The chart that follows demonstrates this phenomenon. It plots the percentage of lean body mass (LBM), which is essentially the weight of the muscles, bones, and organs, and the percentage of body fat as men and women age.

LEAN BODY MASS (LBM) VERSUS FAT, AS WE AGE*

AGE	% LBM	% FAT
	MEN	
25	81	19
50	74	26
70	65	35
	WOMEN	
25	68	32
50	58	42
70	51	49

*Total body weight = 100%.

As you can see, everyone puts on fat with age, even when weight stays the same. You'll also see that the differences between men and women are quite pronounced! A 25-year-old male has more than 80% lean body mass, while a woman of the same age has less than 70%. This difference widens as we age and reflects the fact that men have more natural muscle mass than women. The difference may not seem like that much—13 percentage points or so—but it means that a 175-pound woman who is 50 years old carries almost 30 pounds more fat than a man of the same weight and age, so she's going to have a harder time losing the fat than her husband, who's also overweight. A woman who is 50 has more than 40% body fat. It's just plain harder to lose weight as you get older, especially if you're a woman.

Age aside—and I believe that there should be more leeway given on healthy weights, taking into account the aging process—determining how much you should weigh involves the two factors we've already discussed: health and appearance. Let's deal with the health issue first. At our first meeting, I tell patients my basic rule of thumb about obesity: *You are overweight if you have excess body weight sufficient to impair your health.* The next request I usually get is "At least tell me how much I need to lose so I don't get sick." Answering this is not really that difficult. Suppose a woman weighs 190 pounds, 50 pounds above her ideal weight. If she hasn't contracted any of the three major diseases associated with obesity—cardiovascular disease, diabetes, and hypertension—at that weight, each pound she loses lowers her risk! Her chances of getting one of the "big three" would continue to drop as the weight stayed off. This has been proved in many recent studies, and we will take a closer look at the issue when we learn more about "Syndrome X" in the next chapter.

Now let's take a look at another example: a different woman who also weighs 190 pounds and wants to know how much weight to lose in order to be healthy, but has both high blood pressure and diabetes. My answer to her would be that she should lose the amount of weight that would allow her to maintain normal pressure without medication to regulate her blood pressure. That might be as little as ten pounds. Neither she nor the first woman would have to weigh anywhere near "ideal" body weight in order to be healthier. This new approach to weight is a major message of *The Redux*™ *Revolution.* Redux should work particularly well for both of these women, as we will see.

The cosmetic component of weight loss is more complicated. Each patient who comes into my office fills in a weight-loss questionnaire that asks for detailed information on his or her general health, weight-loss history, and specific medical conditions. Most patients list two "wish" weights on the questionnaire: a "reality" weight, one they truly believe they can attain, and a "fantasy" weight, what they would really like to weigh. The latter is usually based on what they weighed in high school or when they got married, or on the weight of their favorite actor. As I read the questionnaire and examine the patient, I, too, form impressions regarding this individual's two potential weights. Then we compare weights. Rarely are we even in the same ballpark. A 35-year-old, 300-pound man will list 200 pounds as his reality weight and 175 pounds as his fantasy weight. A 45-year-old woman who weighs 220 pounds will tell me that "she'll take" 140–150 pounds, but would really like to be 130 pounds, adding that she has trouble "holding on" at 125 pounds (her college weight of 24 years ago).

These surreal weight-loss expectations may seem innocuous, but they aren't. They have an insidious side to them. I believe them to be remnants of the cult mentality that has been instilled in us by the weight-loss, consumer, and entertainment industries. The subtle—and sometimes unsubtle—message of these industries is that if you can't get down to the weight of a fashion model or television star—and do so pretty quickly—you've lost the weight-loss war (and, in fact, you're probably a loser at the game of life). The message of *The Redux™ Revolution* is different. I don't look at weight loss as a victory or a defeat, but as a skill you can acquire with instruction and practice, like playing the piano. Some people may be better at it than others, but *everyone can do it*!

It takes time and experience to establish this attitude. Usually when people start out, they want to lose a large amount of weight quickly—say, they're at 250 pounds and want to weigh 150. They won't be happy with the modest weight loss, maybe only ten pounds, that we've agreed will make them healthier. When I point out that in order to get to 150 pounds, they've first got to get down to 240 and then 230 and then 220, they tend to be very disappointed at these "paltry" goals, ignoring the difficulty of losing ten pounds and dismissing the achievement that it represents. But once they actually begin to lose weight, their attitude tends to change. I have seen 350-pound women lose ten pounds and feel completely better about themselves. Their entire outlook changes. Often they change their makeup, try a new hairstyle, buy new clothes. Taking off the first ten pounds is a quick way to develop the right attitude, the same attitude that Redux will help you get. Once you finish the book and start the program, your reality weight and your fantasy weight will become welded together.

Many of you seeing the government Optimum Body Weight Ranges chart for the first time may be saying to yourselves, "Maybe I am a bit overweight, but I am not fat. I have a lot of muscle!" Muscle and fat: How much of each do you have? This is important to determine, because your percentage of body fat indicates what your long-term health risk may be. Remember, whenever you step on the scale, you are only measuring body weight, not the percentage of body fat. There are several ways to make this important determination. The least accurate way is the old "pinch" test. In this test, using calipers, skin folds or fat deposits are pinched, and a measurement taken. This can be done at home and is often the method used at health clubs. It does not work! The "gold standard" of body fat measurement is the water immersion test, which is conducted by repeatedly dunking the patient in a pool, over the span of one hour. This is generally done for research purposes and is usually only available in hospitals or research labs.

The self-test method that gives us the most informed reading about our future health is the Body Mass Index (BMI). Essentially, this is an index of how much body fat you have, correlated to your height. It is crucial to know your BMI, because this figure can indicate your risk of developing obesity-related disease. The higher your BMI, the greater your risk. The Federal Drug Administration's guidelines on the use of Redux are based on your knowledge of your BMI, so you had better calculate and know yours. The BMI is hereditary to a certain extent, so by calculating your BMI at a given age, you can calculate your child's probable BMI at that age and know what his or her risk is for future disease. The time to intervene for your health, and your child's, is now.

To calculate your BMI, use the following formula. You will probably need a calculator, because we will be converting inches and pounds to the metric system and squaring numbers. But don't be intimidated; it's easy:

1. Weigh yourself nude, in pounds, and divide your weight by 2.2 (to get kilograms).
2. Measure your height without shoes, in inches, and divide that number by 39.4 (to get your height in meters).
3. Multiply the number you get in Step 2 by itself (that is, square the number).
4. Divide the results of Step 1 by the results of Step 3. This is your BMI.

Here's an example. Let's take the example of the woman who is 5'4" and weighs 185 pounds.

1. 185 divided by 2.2 = 84.
2. 64 inches divided by 39.4 = 1.6.
3. 1.6 x 1.6 = 2.56.
4. 84 divided by 2.56 = 32.8.

This woman's BMI is 32.8. She is at high risk for obesity-related disease. Are you? In order to figure out what level of risk your BMI represents, use the chart that follows.

BMI RISK SCALE

20–25: normal, healthy weight—no great risk
26–29: moderate overweight—moderate risk
30–39: severe overweight—high risk
40 and over: morbid obesity—highest risk

Knowing your BMI is as important as knowing your cho lesterol count or your blood pressure. The good news is that as your BMI goes down, so do your chances for developing obesity-related disease.

Every 60 seconds a person dies in this country from an obesity-related disease, such as diabetes. There are 11 million obese adult-onset diabetics in this country. Diabetes is especially rampant in the African-American and Hispanic communities, where it strikes one person in 20. Obesity itself is even considered a disease by some researchers.

Of course, not all overweight people are unhealthy, but my own experience and my years in practice have persuaded me that anyone who is overweight can look better and be healthier by tapping into some of nature's most intimate secrets. With *The Redux™ Revolution*, you will soon be on the cutting edge of weight-loss knowledge and technology. You will have the answers to questions like:

- Is being overweight really hereditary?
- What factors prevent me from losing weight?
- Why doesn't exercise help me to lose weight?
- Why am I always hungry?
- What can I do to lose weight permanently?

In very short order you will come face to face with the new findings in science that address these questions and many more, and show how Redux may put you on a path to better health. However, in order to fully understand and appreciate this new drug, you must first understand the variations in the human body that help explain why some people are predisposed to being heavy, while others are thin.

DID YOU KNOW . . .

- Each year, 80 million Americans go on a diet.
- The prevalence of obesity doubles between the ages of 20 and 50.
- 50% of African-American and Hispanic women are overweight.
- 50% of all obese children and 75% of all obese adolescents will grow up to be obese adults.
- $60 billion a year is spent on weight loss.
- The average 50-year-old man has a lower percentage of body fat than the average 25-year-old woman.

- There are 15–20 million overweight teens.
- Humans are the only mammals that can voluntarily lose weight.
- In a recent study of nine-year-olds in San Francisco, 40% were dieting.

Chapter 2

Designer Genes

It was 11:00 P.M. on a Saturday night. I was catching the late news before turning in for the night, watching Maria Shriver deliver the latest reports of political disasters and weather-related mayhem. It was the usual late-night newscast, and as I listened to Maria, noting her dark, striking cat's eyes and high, sculpted cheekbones, my mind started to wander. News is news, but the camera loves Maria, angular face and all. She and her husband, Arnold Schwarzenegger, make a very handsome couple, since she is lean and beautiful and he is muscular and toned.

The part of the brain that makes connections between ideas is usually asleep by 11:00 P.M., but this late Saturday night, my brain was working overtime! Wait a minute—those high cheekbones, that lean body. Maria Shriver, I realized, was thin, really thin. I remembered all the pictures I'd seen of her mother, Eunice, with the rest of the "Kennedy sisters," smiling proudly at some political event for brother John or Bobby, or looking sad at a funeral. In those pictures, Eunice and her sisters are thin, very thin. Eunice's mother, Kennedy clan matriarch Rose, who died at age 102, was also thin, and so are most of the other Kennedys I've ever seen pictures of.

My brain was still whirling, and another, very different family popped into my mind. That very week, a family of four from Westchester County, New York, had come to my office for a consultation. To protect their privacy, I will omit their initials and biographical information. The father, in his 30s, weighed 412 pounds. The mother, also in her 30s, weighed 286. The daughter, age 15, weighed 270, and the son, barely 12, tipped the scales at 205. The average weight of this family was almost equal to the average weight of the New York Giants' "front four," and this included two children! Meeting with them was an overwhelming experience, and a sad one. They were all desperate to lose weight and keep it off, and they were devastated by how difficult it was for them to do so. I knew that without help, the children would probably grow up to be even heavier than their parents. I also knew that the fate of the children and their health rested in the hands of their parents, who themselves were at a loss as to what to do.

A Tale of Two Families and Two Genetic Codes

This is truly a tale of two families and two genetic codes! By passing on their "thin" genes to their progeny, the Kennedy parents ensured that their children would be thin. Maria's body is predisposed to be thin, and it is very unlikely that she would be heavy. Just as some people have to put a great deal of effort into being thin, the Kennedys might have to actually put effort into being heavy!

The Westchester County family who came to me for consultation do not fare as well in the gene department. Their genes ordain that they will be heavy. Do not for a moment entertain the idea that if the heavy family ate like the Kennedys, they would be thin like the Kennedys. As we have discussed, the bodies of the overweight are different—and work differently—from the bodies of thin people! The overweight family did not choose to be this way. It is not their "fault" that they are heavy, any more than it is the Kennedys' "fault" that they are thin. This is nature, and nature is sometimes unfair. In this case, nature has ordained that the family from Westchester will be at risk for major health problems—and that even if they can take weight off, they'll have trouble keeping it off. As we'll see, Redux can be of great help to people like this, making an unfair situation seem less unfair.

Two years ago, in 1994, in one of the great medical discoveries of our time, a certain gene was isolated by Dr. Jeffrey Friedman of Rockefeller University. This gene, which affects obesity, is active in slightly overweight people as well as in heavier people. Dr. Friedman's work has caused an explosion in the field of weight loss, the ripples of which will undoubtedly affect you. Redux is the first ripple.

Of Mice and Men

Many of you have seen the television coverage of the scientists working with mice that, bred to lack a certain hormone, became thin. The implications of this for humans were tremendous, because the obesity gene in humans is almost identical to that in mice! The media trumpeted this missing hormone as the breakthrough scientists had been searching for and suggested that a cure for obesity was at hand. The media were half right. These mice had a mutation in their so-called obesity gene, a defect that would not allow them to secrete a chemical that would make them thin. The chemical is leptin. It was hoped that the same gene mutation would be found in obese humans. If this were the case, then giving leptin to overweight humans would have the same dramatic effect it did on the mice—almost immediate loss of body fat. Unfortunately, for now, the obesity gene mutation has not yet been found in humans, so leptin will probably not help humans lose weight, but this could change with further research.

Now, I'll wager that most of you are not concerned with weight loss in rodents, so we'll keep this discussion focused on humans! It's important to understand, though, that the breakthrough science had been waiting for did arrive with those mice: a better understanding of the human obesity gene, paving the way for the Redux Revolution.

Fitting into Your Genes

We've been talking a lot about genetics, and we'll be continuing that discussion, so a review of basic scientific information is in order here. A gene is essentially a piece of DNA (deoxyribonucleic acid), which provides the code for human life. DNA dictates the everyday functions of all the cells in the body, including reproduction. There are thousands of human genes, and genes are present in every living cell, including blood, brain, and heart cells. We all have genes that are unique to us as individuals and can serve forensic or legal medicine as a genetic fingerprint. Our genes tell our cells what substances to make in order to ensure their survival. These required substances include structural proteins, the very building blocks of our bodies. They also include hormones. It's important to recognize, however, that though we all have lots of genes, not all of them are active, or expressed, at any given time. In general, genes are active only when the conditions are right.

The newly discovered obesity gene is no different. The obesity gene makes the leptin found in every fat cell. These cells gather together to form lobules, which then coalesce and form the sheets of fat that we feel when we pinch our abdomens, thighs, and buttocks. We hardly think of them as having a life, but fat cells are very much alive. In heavy people, the obesity gene inside fat cells is very active! It not only manufactures the hormone leptin, which as we shall see plays a role in keeping people heavy, but it also ensures that the next generation that receives the obesity gene will be heavy as well. Now we can understand why the whole family from Westchester County is obese, as well as why the Kennedy family is not. The Kennedys may have the obesity gene, but it is not active, or expressed, in them, while it is extremely active in that family from Westchester County! There is something about the conditions in the fat cells of members of that family—perhaps some malfunction—that makes the conditions right for the obesity gene to be very active.

The fact that obesity has a genetic basis has been known for years. The old saying that the person you marry will eventually look like your in-laws is very true. Many heavy families have children that become heavy at an early age. Let's look at the statistics we discussed in Chapter 1: If you have two parents who are overweight, your chance of being overweight is 80%. With one overweight parent, your chance slips to 40%.

Compare this to having two parents who are not overweight: In that case, your chance of being overweight is just 10%.

But now, with the beginning of the Redux Revolution, we finally have the tools to move in for a closer look at the genetic basis of obesity.

Twin Towers of Success

Studies done with twins have provided a great deal of evidence regarding the genetic basis of obesity, because it's easier to assess the genetic influences on twins than on the average individual. To illustrate this, let's look at S.D. and T.N., two medical technologists in their 40s. They are often asked to participate in university health studies because they are both overweight, they are identical twins, and they are African-American women. Obesity, diabetes, and hypertension are present in 45% of African-American women over 50, and researchers are trying to determine to what degrees genetics and cultural eating practices contribute to their being overweight.

During the course of a number of university-sponsored health studies, S.D. and T.N. were asked to follow various high-protein and low-fat diets and exercise plans. They were studied individually, and sometimes together. They were given extensive blood tests and had their metabolic rates tested using the highly acclaimed water-immersion technique mentioned in Chapter 1. They lost weight during the studies and gained it back between studies. This constant "yo-yoing" did not allow for weight loss; in fact, though they'd been dieting under close supervision, their weight continued to creep upward.

When they came into my office for help with weight loss, S.D. weighed 190 pounds and T.N. weighed 184 pounds. I started each on two medications, phentermine and fenflura-mine, a regimen that will be discussed in Chapter 8. In one month, S.D.'s weight went down to 183 pounds and T.N.'s went to 178 pounds. I saw them both, together, every three weeks, charting their progress with weight and health, but never discussing food or dietary regimens with them. By the end of the second month, S.D. dropped to 176 pounds and T.N. to 174. Incidentally, these two women do not live to-gether, have separate families, and do not share meals often. This pattern of weighing within just a few pounds of each other continued, to my amazement. Today, S.D. weighs 154 pounds and T.N. weighs 151. They have had a parallel weight-loss experience. After seven months of the same treat-ment—but different eating regimens and life experiences—they weigh almost exactly the same. Since their bodies have responded to different environments in the same fashion, we must conclude that they have identical internal reasons for losing weight in such similar patterns. The lessons that these fascinating women have taught us are:

- Appetite is often inherited.
- Even though they both have the obesity gene, they both "outsmarted" their genes—and so can you. This can happen if you just listen to the message that your body is trying to tell you, the message found in the newly discovered "fat hor-mone," leptin.

Leptin—Is It Greek to You?

Leptin—from the Greek word *leptos*, meaning "thin"—is the hormone manufactured by the obesity gene in the fat cells. Hormones are chemical messengers that send information from a gland or group of cells to other parts of the body. Leptin is the fat-cell hormone. The greater the percentage of body fat (the higher your BMI, remember?), the more leptin your body produces. Leptin travels through the bloodstream until it reaches an area of the brain called the hypothalamus. Our appetite control center is located in this marble-sized structure, which plays an important role in regulating appetite and weight loss.

When the body is working as it should, leptin tells the brain when we have adequate stores of fat. The brain, in turn, reacts to this message by shutting down the appetite center and keeping a record of how much fat is being stored. When there is an "adequate" amount of fat in our bodies, the brain is satisfied and no hunger signals are sent out. All of this happens via two middlemen, the neurotransmitters (or nerve messengers) galanin and neuropeptide Y. First described by Dr. Sarah Leibowitz in a 1992 paper based on her earlier work as a researcher at the Rockefeller University in New York, these are two tiny protein substances that control our appetite for various nutrients. Together they control our appetite for predominantly high-fat and high-carbohydrate foods—which, incidentally, are two of the main components of the American fast-food diet. Of the two, it seems that neuropeptide Y is the more important player. Studies have shown that when the level of neuropeptide Y in the hypothalamus is high, food intake is increased and fat deposits are promoted. When the level of neuropeptide Y is low, food intake decreases and the body lays down less fat for storage. Normally, a high level of leptin keeps the level of neuropeptide Y down. This hormonal exchange has been verified in mice and is presumed to work the same way in humans.

However, this mechanism is somehow defective in the obese! In people who are obese, leptin levels are high, but neuropeptide Y levels are high as well, when they should be lower, as is the case in thinner individuals. It is the leptin/neuropeptide Y ratio that drives the need to eat. If you are overweight, your desire to eat is increased via this mechanism. The obesity gene makes leptin, but leptin does not give the proper signal to the brain to shut off production of neuropeptide Y. Neuropeptide Y makes you eat and increase your fat stores. Amazingly, your genes and even your own brain are working against you! I told you that being heavy isn't your fault! When we understand this, the Redux Revolution gains momentum.

Furthermore, neuropeptide Y is very sensitive to starvation and exercise. What happens when a heavy person starves himself and starts to deplete the body's fat stores? The brain signals the body to eat, so more fat is stored. What happens when a heavy person exercises? As you'll see, when we answer this question, we are going to extend the weight-loss revolution even further.

Rats! I Didn't Know That

A study done in Liverpool, England, gives us an important insight into the effects of exercise. In fact, I'd venture to say that this research may have the same impact on your weight loss that another import from Liverpool had on your musical tastes in 1964. The researchers studied two groups of ten rats each. They had one group exercise heavily. The second group had their food intake restricted, so that their weight loss matched that of the first group, but they were not made to exercise.

After 40 days, the scientists measured the levels of neuropeptide Y in both groups. Amazingly, both groups had identically elevated levels of neuropeptide Y. The rats' brains interpreted the loss of calories *by either diet or exercise* as an equal threat to their set point levels, and they tried to counter this by increasing appetite. The "set point" is the body's own internal thermostat. It attempts to keep the body at a given body weight and fights weight loss, as well as weight gain. It accomplishes this by altering metabolism, the rate at which your body "burns" its "fuel"—the food you eat.

We humans owe a great deal to those Liverpudlian rats! They taught us a lesson so important that it will rock the very foundations of our weight-loss culture. Their lesson also helped set the stage for Redux, as we will see in the next chapter. Here's the lesson: People with a very active obesity gene—like you—who go on low-calorie diets and/or exercise vigorously will, like the rats, have elevated levels of neuropeptide Y in the brain. This increase in neuropeptide Y forces them to eat, helps to deposit fat, and leads to weight gain. It might take days, it might take months, but it will happen. *When you go on a diet or exercise vigorously, your own body will sabotage your weight loss!* This explains why diets and exercise fail to cause lasting weight loss in overweight people.

Back to Pencils and Zeppelins

How do you know if you have a very active obesity gene? There is no blood test for this now, but it will probably be easier to test indirectly for the obesity gene by testing for high levels of leptin. This test could be available soon. For the time being, assume that if you are overweight, have a parent who is overweight, or have a grandparent who is overweight, you probably have a very active obesity gene. Keep in mind that you do not have to be grossly overweight to have such a gene.

A beer belly can be a manifestation of an active obesity gene. People with slight degrees of overweight also may have active obesity genes.

There is a quantitative aspect to the functioning of the obesity gene, as well. As we discussed earlier, if you were overweight as a child and have remained overweight during your adult life, you probably have what is known as hyperplastic obesity. This means that you have an increased number of fat cells. Even when you lose weight, the fat cells never disappear; they only tend to shrink in size. For reasons that are as yet unknown, this fact appears to play a role in making it more difficult for hyperplastic people to lose weight. As you may recall from Chapter 1, I call this kind of person a Zeppelin.

Now, a Zeppelin is a balloon, but by no means is it just another blimp. In fact, it's a beautiful, streamlined airship of World War I vintage. If you are a Zeppelin, you can attain a beautiful, streamlined shape, but you will never become a Pencil. Pencils are people without a family history of obesity, and while they may have the obesity gene, it is not very well expressed. Under certain circumstances, these people can still reach very high weights—300 to 400 pounds—but when they are overweight, they also have the biochemical potential to lose weight more easily than Zeppelins. Their type of obesity is called hypertrophic, meaning that though their fat cells may be larger than normal, the number of fat cells they have is within the normal range. Pencils have the potential to be thin permanently. It's downright unfair that obese Pencils can lose more weight more easily than obese Zeppelins, but Redux can make the situation fairer, as we will see in the next chapter.

The Game Is Over

All along you suspected that there was something different about you. Something was going on inside your body, blocking the road to weight-loss success: a genetic biochemical defect. Following is a chart that sums up the struggle that you and your body have been engaged in from the time you went on your first diet. The left column illustrates your efforts. The right column illustrates your body's response, in light of the new research we just discussed.

YOUR DIET	YOUR BODY'S RESPONSE
1. Willpower level is high.	1. Diets based on willpower usually last 45 days.
2. Calorie restriction begins	2. Body begins to lose muscle, even before fat, and senses starvation. Neuropeptide Y levels rise.
3. Weight loss begins.	3. Muscle continues to be lost, the metabolic rate falls, appetite increases.
4. Weight loss peaks after a few weeks.	4. In response to calorie restriction, leptin level falls 50%, neuropeptide Y level is high, appetite is high.
5. Weight loss slows, a plateau is reached, frustration grows.	5. Neuropeptide Y level is high.
6. Diet ends.	6. Appetite stays high and weight is gained, surpassing the starting weight.

Bottom line: You lose the game but not the weight. The body wins a battle it set the rules for anyway! Now we have only one more stop before we meet Redux, which has the power to level the playing field! (If you are interested, a similar chart awaits you later in the book. Except this time, *you* come out the winner.)

"Syndrome X"—Are You X-Rated?

Whether you are 15 pounds overweight or 150 pounds overweight, whether you are a Pencil or a Zeppelin, you may be a "Syndrome X-er," too! As I mentioned in Chapter 1, the discovery of the science behind Syndrome X was one of the scientific breakthroughs that set the stage for the Redux Revolution. Syndrome X is a newly identified medical entity that may explain why millions of people, and perhaps you, are unable to lose weight. If you have Syndrome X, you may very well be on the way to developing one or more of the "big three" medical complications of being overweight: cardiac disease, hypertension, and diabetes.

Stay Away from This Gang

Syndrome X is also known as the "insulin resistance syndrome." It was originally described by Dr. Gerald Reaven of Stanford University and has undergone much revision since his original description in 1988. A syndrome is a group of symptoms that occur together. Syndrome X is a constellation of medical abnormalities that work synergistically to make an overweight person prone to problems in the blood vessels, leading to the "big three."

These abnormalities include, but are not limited to:

- High blood pressure
- High insulin levels
- High cholesterol and low HDL (the "good" cholesterol)
- Abnormal blood-clotting mechanisms (which make blood "thick" and may lead to strokes)
- Abnormal blood sugar responses (tending toward diabetes)
- High triglycerides (a type of fat found in the blood)
- Insulin resistance (explained below)

These are all major risk factors for cardiovascular disease. These abnormalities can also be found in thin persons, but they are far more common in people who are overweight. You can have one, all, or any combination. And, though we know these are serious risk factors, there is no single defining blood test that clinches the diagnosis.

Some researchers believe that if you have an increased waist/hip ratio—that is, if you are apple-shaped, and your abdomen is wider than your hips—you will suffer more from the consequences of Syndrome X. It is believed that excess fat around the abdomen behaves differently, biochemically speaking, from fat in other parts of the body. This abdominal fat is more likely to raise blood pressure and increase atherosclerosis—a condition of fatty plaque buildup in the arteries leading to increased risk of heart attack and stroke. Perhaps pear-shaped people (those with wider hips than abdomen, the "bottom-heavy" people of life) fare better, but a recent study from Canada shows that they have subtle biochemical problems that may put them at greater risk for cardiovascular disease than was previously thought.

For our discussion, the important things to know are:

• Having Syndrome X puts you at an extremely high risk of developing coronary heart disease and diabetes.
• Syndrome X has a genetic component.
• Syndrome X is self-perpetuating: Once you have any of its components, they remain and may get progressively worse, unless weight loss occurs.

Syndrome X can be controlled with weight loss, yet its genetic component makes weight loss difficult—even impossible, as we've discussed. Until now. It is very important that you understand Syndrome X because Redux has tremendous potential to control it! Using Redux can actually improve all the factors we've just listed.

The unifying factor of the different components of Syndrome X is insulin resistance, a key concept in understanding obesity and adult-onset diabetes, which are intimately related.

Is Your Resistance High?

Insulin is a hormone that controls the fate of the carbohydrates (sugars) you eat and, indirectly, of certain dietary fats as well. Under normal circumstances, when the body is working well, levels of insulin, which is manufactured in the pancreas, rise in response to a sugar load in the blood—that is, generally in response to your eating. Insulin's function is to keep the blood sugar level on an even keel, even after a meal. After its work of pushing blood sugar into the muscles and the fat cells is completed—again, this is only under normal conditions—insulin is shooed offstage by a counterregulatory hormone called glucagon. Glucagon then tends to raise the level of sugar in the blood. About three hours after a carbohydrate-containing meal, insulin begins to reach its basal (lowest) level.

In addition to regulating sugar levels in the blood, insulin also plays a role in the metabolism of fat: The presence of insulin makes it easier for your body to store fat. Even more important to our Redux discussion, insulin is the chief hormone that promotes hunger! The more insulin you have circulating in your body, the hungrier you are! Guess what overweight people have? You've got it—lots of insulin, a condition called hyperinsulinemia. This is due to a condition called insulin resistance. Somehow, the muscles, or even fat itself, block the insulin from doing its job correctly. As a result, blood sugar levels rise ever so slightly above normal and stay there, all the time. When the body senses this rise in blood sugar, it tells the pancreas to make more insulin. This cycle continues, and as more insulin is secreted into the blood, hunger is stimulated and weight gain ensues. Pitting a measly diet against this highly sophisticated weight-retaining mechanism is a "Custer's Last Stand" of weight loss. Even if you lose a few pounds in a couple of weeks or months, your elevated insulin levels will eventually catch up to you and you will regain the weight. The body's biochemical willpower always outlasts your willpower.

The heavier you are, the more insulin resistance you have. Your insulin levels are always elevated, and they rise even more right after you eat. The more insulin resistance and hyperinsulinemia you have, the hungrier you will be. Insulin resistance is often already present in the children of parents who are diabetics and hypertensives. This further strengthens the idea of the hereditary nature of obesity.

Bottom line: If you have a family history of obesity, you may have high insulin levels and insulin resistance, both components of Syndrome X—which means you need to come up with a new, smarter way to lose weight.

Zapping the X

Weight loss lowers all of the risk factors of Syndrome X. Recent research has indicated that Redux has a beneficial effect on these risk factors, *independent* of weight loss. In other words, Redux works against Syndrome X itself! This is very good news for the overweight people I see who know they're genetically at risk for cardiovascular disease but who have felt helpless to prevent it. I believe that this application of Redux will be among its most important uses, particularly since not much weight loss is needed in order to lower the risk factors of Syndrome X. With Redux, perhaps it's goodbye, Syndrome X!

Obesity genes, leptin, neuropeptide Y, Syndrome X— these are powerful internal forces that have been opposing your weight-loss efforts. It's as if your body has made a great deal of effort to create special metabolic pathways in order to maintain itself at an increasingly heavier weight.

But all is not lost. Remember the story of the twin medical technicians? They both lost weight because they not only outsmarted their obesity genes, they actually tricked their brains into allowing them to get thin. With the help of Redux, you will be given the same chance!

DID YOU KNOW . . .

- A pound of fat has the volume of a softball.
- A pound of muscle has the volume of a hardball.
- The average diet lasts 45 days.
- Every 60 seconds, another person is diagnosed with diabetes.
- Average cholesterol levels have gone down in the last decade, but average weight has gone up.
- The average American woman is 5'4" and weighs 144 pounds.
- The average American female model is 5'7" and weighs 115–120 pounds.

Chapter 3

Redux to the Rescue

In every culture, there is some kind of quest—to find peace, to find knowledge, to find love, to find power. For example, the ancients took it upon themselves to try to locate the human soul. Each successive civilization has tried to trace its anatomical locale. The Babylonians believed the home of the soul was the heart. The Greeks thought it was the liver, and the Aztecs thought it was in the blood.

In our culture, much attention has been paid to locating the actual site that controls our appetite, perhaps because our human appetites seem to be out of control so much of the time! About 250 years ago, we started to zero in on the very place where appetite is controlled: the brain. In *Primitive Physick*, a small book written by John Wesley, A.M. (the founder of Methodism), and published in London in 1763, a possible cure for binge eating was suggested. At that time, binge eating was called "canine appetite," which was described as "an insatiable appetite of eating." The Reverend Mr. Wesley suggested that a small bit of bread dipped in wine and applied to the nostrils would stop a binge. Mediating a binge via the nostrils is not as far-fetched as it might seem, since the olfactory bulb, the part of the nose involved with the sense of smell, which stimulates appetite, is actually an outcropping of the brain itself.

Each new discovery in the field of weight loss has suggested that the brain is the location of the appetite control center. During the past century, it has become apparent that the epicenter of appetite control is located in a small, marble-sized structure in the brain called the hypothalamus.

You have already been introduced to the hypothalamus, leptin, and neuropeptide Y in Chapter 2. Now let's take a brief overview of cerebral anatomy and physiology so you'll have all the information you need to make sense of the Redux Revolution.

The brain can be divided into two parts: the higher, or upper, part of the brain, known as the cerebral hemispheres, and the lower parts of the brain, which encompass the cerebellum, the medula oblongata, and the brain stem. The brain also has a hierarchy of functions, known, conveniently enough, as the higher and lower. Higher functions, which include thinking, reasoning, decision-making, and speech, are performed by the two halves of the upper part of the brain, or the cerebral cortex. The lower functions, which include processing sensory information from the environment, governing locomotion, and regulating actions of the reflexes, take place in several different places, one of them being the brain stem. The hypothalamus, which mediates and coordinates between higher and lower functions, is located right below the cerebral hemispheres, in an area called the midbrain.

The hypothalamus functions as a central relay station to the rest of the body and other parts of the brain. Not only does this tiny structure contain our appetite center, but it also plays a huge role in controlling moods, body temperature, ability to experience pleasure (including sexual pleasure), and sleep. In addition, it plays a part in our ability to perceive punishment and reward. The hypothalamus contains nerve cells that tell us when we must eat and when we are full and should stop eating. These cells are part of the system of interconnected nerve fibers that send and receive information from the far reaches of the body and other parts of the brain. This information exists in the form of a biochemical signal, made up of neurotransmitters. Neurotransmitters trigger the brain to send out its own electrical signals. These signals constitute the brain's activities, from thinking to making it possible to sleep.

A Piece of Cake

To visualize how the brain and body interact, imagine that a piece of chocolate cake is placed in front of you. First the higher parts of the cerebral cortex must verify that it is indeed a piece of chocolate cake. The brain receives the sensory information it needs from your eyes, your nose, and, if you touch the cake, your fingers. The signal that reaches the cortex from the nerve endings in your eyes, nose, or fingers is transmitted via the neurotransmitters. Keep in mind that this entire process occurs in mere milliseconds! Once the brain has come to the conclusion that this is indeed a piece of chocolate cake, a more important issue arises: Should you eat it or not? The cortex now sends a quick message to the hypothalamus. This message is to determine if you are already physically satisfied or instead "need" the extra calories of the cake; if you need the taste sensation of the cake to help your mood; or if you have the need to feel full or pampered. This message is also sent via neurotransmitters. Notice that a question can be conscious—"Are you in the mood for chocolate cake?"—or unconscious—"Does your body need the calories?" The appetite center in the hypothalamus is now carrying the ball. In addition to answering these questions, it must decide if you should eat the cake. It checks the internal memory circuits: "Is this Aunt Rose's cake, the one you love, or is this the local supermarket variety, the one that gave you diarrhea the last time you ate it?" The hypothalamus must also check with your stomach, to see if it's full or not. Now a new question is posed: "Are you hungry or not?" Finally, a decision is reached. The hypothalamus has notified the brain that you are hungry, that the appetite center is not satisfied, and that Aunt Rose's chocolate cake will remedy the situation. And all of this checking, evaluating, and decision-making takes place in the amount of time it takes for the salivary glands in your mouth to start watering. Go ahead and eat the cake!

But now let's suppose that you've been through this process many times, and you've always eaten the cake, with the result that you're now 40 pounds overweight. Wouldn't it be wonderful if you could somehow have the hypothalamus tell the other parts of the brain that you are full and do not need the chocolate cake? Wouldn't it be great if those hunger signals that travel from the stomach to the hypothalamus could be blunted?

Chemical Reaction

This is exactly how Redux works! It alters the biochemical signals so that the appetite center in the hypothalamus is tricked into thinking that you are not hungry and that you are satisfied. The signal is the neurotransmitter serotonin. There are many chemicals in the brain that qualify as neurotransmitters, or chemical messengers. These include dopamine, which is involved in the perception of reality and plays a role in the development of Parkinson's disease; noradrenaline, which is involved in the ability to pay attention; and serotonin, which is involved in feeding. Serotonin also plays a role with regard to depression, mood swings, aggression, and anxiety.

Serotonin is among the chief neurotransmitters of the hypothalamus. It is an extremely powerful chemical, packing an amazing punch. When scientists study serotonin, the amounts they work with are measured in nanograms. A nanogram is roughly one ten-billionth of a pound! When it comes to hunger, the actions of serotonin seem very straightforward: When serotonin levels in the hypothalamus are high, you are not hungry, and when they are low, you are hungry. Redux blocks the process by which serotonin is reabsorbed into a nerve after it communicates with another nerve—the process called re-uptake. When serotonin re-uptake is blocked by Redux, serotonin does not enter the cell. Instead, it accumulates outside the cell in the empty spaces between nerve endings, called the synapses. This accumulation causes a total increase in the amount of serotonin in the hypothalamus. The elevation of serotonin levels shuts off the appetite center and can also cause an elevation in mood.

Serotonin itself contains the amino acid tryptophan. Amino acids are the building blocks of proteins. Tryptophan is one of the nine "essential" amino acids—ones the body cannot manufacture but must absorb from the diet. So we must take in tryptophan from food. High-carbohydrate meals have been shown to elevate levels of tryptophan and serotonin in the brain. Some researchers have advocated eating meals that are high in protein and high in carbohydrate because such meals lead to increased levels of serotonin in the brain and will shut off appetite. I strongly recommend not eating this way, since producing excess tryptophan, as a result of eating high-carbohydrate, high-protein meals, can promote drowsiness, which is a high price to pay when you're trying to shut down the appetite center. More important, though, is the fact that eating is a personal experience. Telling you what you "should" eat or not eat to lose weight is overcontrolling—it's downright dictatorial—and it doesn't work. The whole idea behind taking Redux, as we shall see in Chapter 5, is that you should be able to lose weight on *your own* diet—not someone else's!

In our chocolate cake example, you may recall that the hypothalamus monitored signals from its own appetite center and from the stomach. Hunger and appetite, while closely related, are not the same thing. Hunger is the visceral sensation that tells you it's time to eat. The gnawing feeling in the stomach, the sensation of weakness—that's hunger. The message of hunger is clear: The body needs food and you had better eat!

Appetite is the *subjective desire* to eat. It relates to a higher, more "civilized" approach to food than hunger. It includes our ability to enjoy food and refine our eating habits. Signals for both hunger and appetite are filtered in the hypothalamus. Redux reduces both hunger and appetite because the com-

mon pathway both use to get to the hypothalamus is serotonin. However, you don't have to worry that by taking
Redux you will be giving control of yourself to an outside
power, the way marijuana was presented as working in the
classic film warning against drug use, *Reefer Madness,* or as
many people who have taken diet pills (amphetamines) have
experienced.

With Redux, you're in control, not the drug. Although
the hypothalamus makes recommendations regarding appetite
and hunger—and sometimes very strong recommendations
indeed—the cerebral cortex has the final call and is the ultimate controller of both hunger and appetite. Evidence of this
can be seen in the fact that even the hungriest overweight
person can observe a fast, rather than eat, for religious reasons
or before surgery. This is because the cortex is responsible for
all food judgments, in terms of intake, and is closely associated
with discipline, a fact that is highly pertinent to the use of
Redux. Since Redux works at the hypothalamus level, not
in the cortex, it cannot overwhelm you and assume control.
You always have control over Redux because your cortex,
with its higher functioning, still reigns supreme.

Revolution on the Mood Front

In addition to influencing our food intake, serotonin also
takes part in determining what kind of mood we're in, what
our level of anxiety is, and whether we need sleep. Some of
the side effects of Redux that we will examine in the next
chapter are based on the intimate anatomical relationship that
anchors these factors in the hypothalamus. For instance, a
slight imbalance in the amount of serotonin involved in the
sleep center of the hypothalamus can cause increased sleepi-

ness, which is a known side effect of Redux. This implies that Redux's influence is not limited to the appetite center. Future drugs of this type may be.

However, there is also a favorable consequence of all these factors being "sardined" in the hypothalamus. This positive result has to do with the control of binge and emotional eating. Often people overeat out of depression or emotional upset. It has been proved that these emotional states are related to having low levels of serotonin in the brain.

In fact, as we'll soon see, the Redux Revolution was made possible by the development of a whole generation of antidepressants that work by raising the level of serotonin in the brain. These drugs are called selective serotonin re-uptake inhibitors (SSRIs), and fluoxetine, sold under the trade name Prozac, is the prototype. One of the benefits of the revolution is that by keeping the level of serotonin elevated, Redux can prevent bingeing, or at least lessen the amount of food consumed. As a by-product, Redux can also keep mood elevated.

Future research will try to determine what effect, if any, serotonin has on neuropeptide Y. You will recall from the previous chapter that neuropeptide Y is another key player in increasing appetite. It also acts in the hypothalamus, receiving messages from the fat cells throughout the body via the hormone leptin. We've noted that the leptin–neuropeptide Y axis does not work properly in obese individuals. At this point, we do not know whether Redux has some inhibitory action on neuropeptide Y. We will have to wait for this answer.

For now, we know that Redux works. We know how Redux works. But the most important question is: Does Redux help overweight patients take off the weight? To find the answer, let's look at a bit of pharmaceutical history.

The European Experience

Although it is new to the United States, Redux has been used for over ten years in more than 60 countries in Europe and Asia and in Australia. The development of Redux started in the late 1970s, when clinical studies noted a link between levels of serotonin and the eating disorder called bulimia, commonly characterized by episodes of bingeing and purging—eating copious amounts of food and then vomiting. The bodies of bulimics manufacture lower levels of serotonin than normal and are very sensitive to fluctuations in serotonin. This disorder is associated with depression and, interestingly, 90% of bulimics are young women. During this time, the drug company Eli Lilly was working on a medication to combat bulimia. It came up with Prozac, the well-known antidepressant. Remember, the hypothalamus controls moods, including depression, and Prozac works similarly to Redux: It keeps levels of serotonin high in the brain. This elevates mood and does not permit the fluctuations in serotonin levels that can cause mood swings.

As with many great discoveries in medicine, some of the spin-offs are even more remarkable than the initial discovery. As clinical trials of Prozac continued, it was noticed that one of Prozac's side effects was weight loss. Further research by other groups led to the development of a drug called fenfluramine (Pondimin), which also works by keeping serotonin levels high and depressing appetite. It was found to be safe and effective and was approved for use in this country two decades ago. Today it is used in the phen/fen (phentermine/fenfluramine) regime that is detailed later in this book. Further experiments with fenfluramine showed that if you change the configuration of the molecule (its chemical structure), you can increase its potency and decrease its side effects. This led to the development of dexfenfluramine—Redux!

Some of the early research that led to the development of Redux is most interesting. For instance, scientists discovered a method by which they could measure the link between stress and eating. They would pinch the tails of rats, which would induce the rats to eat. It was found that if the scientists pinched the rats' tails repeatedly, the rats became so stressed that they became obese! The next discovery in this study was that if the rats were given a particular drug prior to the tail pinching, they would not eat nearly as much as they would if their tails were pinched without the medication. The medication was fenfluramine! This was one of the first forms of proof that fenfluramine, along with Redux, can stop binge eating—even when a person is "stressed out"!

Bringing Redux Home

Dexfenfluramine was first made by a French company, Les Laboratoires Servier. The U.S. patent for dexfenfluramine was acquired by Drs. Richard and Judith Wurtman of the Massachusetts Institute of Technology. In 1993, the company that the Wurtmans formed, Interneuron, petitioned the FDA to introduce the drug in the United States. As is the standard procedure, the petition from Interneuron first went to an advisory committee at the FDA for study. Originally, the FDA's advisory committee recommended that dexfenfluramine not be released in the United States because of concern involving a study conducted in 1994. In this study, animals that were given high doses of the drug showed brain damage. (There was also concern about the possibility of a serious lung disorder developing as the result of taking dexfenfluramine, a matter we will address in Chapter 4.)

However, after a follow-up to the Johns Hopkins study was done by scientists at the Environmental Protection Agency, which found that dexfenfluramine caused no brain damage, Interneuron's petition was back on track at the FDA. After reviewing the results of clinical trials involving some 4,500 patients (900 of whom were in the United States), on November 17, 1995, the FDA advisory committee recommended release of Redux for use in the United States by a six-to-five vote.

In a press release, Glenn L. Cooper, M.D., president and chief executive officer of Interneuron, said: "Redux is now positioned to become the first obesity drug approved for long-term use in this country." The advisory committee's decision was not the final one, however. Full FDA approval was still pending. It should be mentioned that Dr. Henry Bine, of the Henry Ford Hospital in Detroit and chairman of the advisory committee at the time of the decision, voted against the drug's release in the United States. He felt there wasn't enough information available on the drug's long-term safety.

On April 29, 1996, the FDA approved Redux for use in the United States. Redux is marketed by American Home Products and is currently manufactured by Wyeth-Ayerst. Upon approving the drug, the FDA noted that the brain damage cited earlier was not found in humans and that the pulmonary problems that had been of concern are very rare. Dr. James Bilstad, of the FDA's division of metabolic drugs, which had been responsible for the review of all the data associated with Redux, said that "the benefits outweigh the risks."

The FDA has not placed a time restriction on how long patients can use Redux. It is important to know that no studies using Redux have extended for longer than one year. This is a key point that we will examine more closely.

The Redux™ Revolution is committed to making you the most informed consumer on the pros and cons of Redux. If you decide to take Redux, you must be an informed consumer and work closely with your health professional. What follows is a review of the major worldwide studies used to establish Redux's efficiency. These are the same studies reviewed by the FDA and used in making the decision to approve Redux. Now you can read about them and decide for yourself whether Redux may be for you.

Putting Redux to the Test

In petitioning the FDA for Redux's release, Interneuron provided a review of 17 different studies on Redux; in addition, the FDA scientists had scores of supporting studies to review. In the studies submitted by Interneuron, the average age of the patients was 41 years, and 82% were females. They averaged a BMI (Body Mass Index; see Chapter 1) of 34, and their average weight was about 204 pounds. Sixteen of the 17 studies were carried out for three months. All but one showed statistically significant weight loss. The studies included different diet protocols, drawn up by the universities and hospitals that performed the research, so the conclusion can be drawn that the Redux, and not the specific diet, was what contributed to the weight loss.

One large, long-term study was entitled "International Trial of Long-Term Dexfenfluramine in Obesity" and is commonly referred to as the "Index" study. It was conducted by Dr. Bernard Guy-Grand et al. and appeared in 1989 in the prestigious British medical journal the *Lancet*. The study included 822 patients from five countries: England, France, Italy, Belgium, and Germany. The patients were randomly assigned to one of two groups. One group received Redux, the other received a placebo disguised as Redux. Neither the investigators nor the patients knew who was receiving which pill, making this a "double-blind" experiment. Patients ranged in age from 18 to 75, and all had BMIs over 30, which meant they were at risk for cardiovascular disease. There were four times as many women as men in this study. Various calorie-restricting diets, none lower than 1,450 calories, were instituted, including one using guidelines from Weight Watchers. Patients were followed for one year, and during that time, 41 patients dropped out because of clinical problems with the side effects of Redux, and 38 patients who were receiving placebo dropped out.

Of the patients who completed the study, those who had taken Redux lost 33% to 55% more weight than those in the control groups—who had lost weight as well. Most patients' weight loss peaked at six months and then slowed. About 100 patients lost 30% of their initial body weight. This is the equivalent of a 300-pound person losing 90 pounds! Most patients had more modest weight loss. The actual numbers looked like this:

• Eight out of ten patients taking Redux lost four pounds within the first month of trial.
• Six out of ten of this original 80% went on to lose significant body weight within the next 12 months.

Interestingly, patients who did not lose the initial 4 pounds within the first month of trial had a 90% chance of failing to lose significant weight over the next 12 months. The result of this study favorable to adherents of Redux was that *only the patients on Redux were able to keep the weight off.* This finding is of key importance. It means that some measure of fairness and equity has been established at last for Zeppelins and Pencils: With Redux, once the weight drops off, it stays off, no matter what your genetic heritage! The researchers involved in the study believed, based on an extrapolation of their data, that the same results could be attained by the general public.

Another study, by H. T. O'Conner et al., published in the *International Journal of Obesity and Related Metabolic Disorders* in 1995, also showed that Redux doubled the amount of total weight loss achieved by diet alone.

Now we'll show some actual weight-loss numbers. After three months, the weight loss from all studies ranged from a high of 23 pounds to five pounds. Keep in mind, this involved patients taking a pill and consuming a diet of no less than 1,450 calories, which means that no study involved drastic low-caloric diets. About 6% of the patients had to discontinue Redux because of its side effects, and half of these patients suffered serious side effects, such as severe fatigue, diarrhea, or headaches. Believe it or not, however, many members of the placebo group, who received disguised sugar pills, had about the same amount of side effects as the Redux group! In fact, these individuals actually often experienced more serious side effects and had to stop taking the placebo pill!

Based on these studies, Interneuron reached the following conclusions:

• Redux works to cut appetite and reduce weight.
• Changing the accompanying diet has no effect on Redux's efficiency.
• Redux was well tolerated.
• A four-pound weight loss after one month on Redux predicted a successful weight loss after one year on Redux.

It's also notable that, given the range of studies, it's clear that both Pencils and Zeppelins were able to lose weight with Redux. Moreover, Redux may augment weight loss for overweight individuals who have achieved some weight loss by dieting alone: According to the manufacturer, among obese patients who had been successful in losing weight by dieting alone (i.e., lost at least 10 pounds in the prior year), the addition of Redux to the regimen resulted in the further loss of 26% of initial excess weight.

An interesting Dutch study by R. Voelker was featured in a 1995 issue of the *International Journal of Obesity and Related Metabolic Disorders*. Like the "Index" study mentioned earlier, this study divided moderately obese patients into two groups: one taking Redux, the other taking a placebo disguised as Redux. Each group was given one-quarter of their normal daily diet in the form of heavy-carbohydrate foods and high-fat snacks. They could eat as much as they wanted, so if a person was accustomed to eating 4,000 calories a day, he or she could eat 1,000 of them in snacks! It was found that Redux lowered the amount of food eaten at meals, as well as the amount of high-carbohydrate foods and high-fat snacks consumed. Moreover, people taking Redux lost an average of 6.5 pounds over nine weeks, despite having no dietary restrictions! No one in the placebo group lost weight. (A study published in the same journal two years earlier seemed to demonstrate that Redux may play a role in raising the metabolism after eating. This would make it easier for people who take the drug to lose weight and keep it off over time. However, another, similar study did not agree with this finding, so more research is needed.)

Other studies done in Australia, New Zealand, and Belgium all reached the same conclusion: Redux caused statistically significant weight loss with minimal side effects.

Nonetheless, these studies confirm that when evaluating a drug's efficacy, the gamut of clinical responses can be large. For comparison, let's look at the use of aspirin for relief of headaches. Suppose 1,000 people try it. Of these, 600 may get a good response where the symptoms are fully resolved, 200 may get a partial response and require another medication, and 200 may have no response at all. Who is "right"? They all are. The different responses are due to many factors, including the nature of the headache, tolerability and perception of pain, and expectations of cure vs. control of the medicine. The list of potential variables is large.

The same holds true for Redux. There are so many variables in the causes and treatment of obesity that, as the FDA emphasized upon its approval of the drug, even Redux will not work for everyone. Yet, it worked well enough for the FDA to grant it approval!

It is natural for you to be looking for the way to lose the most weight in the least amount of time, looking for the dramatic successes featured on commercials and in the case examples of most diet books. Remember, some patients lost 50–100 pounds while taking Redux, some lost five! It's important to recognize that the FDA was not looking at how much weight could be lost on Redux, but rather at the total number of people who could lose weight on the drug—especially in light of all the health risks obesity poses. If Redux could cause weight loss in many people, no matter how modest the amount, then it has great potential to be used to prevent some of the dangers of obesity—much as we vaccinate children to safeguard them against common infectious agents.

It turns out that not only can Redux facilitate weight loss in the many people but it has another benefit that was unknown to the original researchers, until recently. Redux has actually been shown to lower cardiac risk factors such as high blood pressure, high insulin levels, elevated cholesterol, and all the other components of Syndrome X. This occurs independent of weight loss, which also lowers cardiac risk factors!

In its approval of Redux, the FDA recognized an exciting possibility: If Redux lowers cardiac risk factors, then can we expect to see an increase in health and longevity and a decrease in deaths related to obesity nationally? Are there studies to help us reach such a powerful conclusion?

Yes—there are many! Including "Dexfenfluramine (Redux) Reduces Cardiovascular Risk Factors," by J. Bremer et al., and "Effect of Dexfenfluramine on Body Weight, Blood Pressure, Insulin Resistance, and Serum Cholesterol in Obese Individuals," by I. Holdaway et al., both published in the respected *International Journal of Obesity and Related Metabolic Disorders*, in 1994 and 1995 respectively. Another study, from the *Medical Journal of Australia* in 1993, entitled "Dexfenfluramine (Redux) in Type II Diabetes: Effect on Weight and Diabetes Control" by G. O. Stewart et al., points the way as well. These carefully done studies show that Redux can actually lower blood pressure, cholesterol, glucose, and insulin levels in the obese, even with only moderate weight loss.

There is even a study in the 1995 issue of *Metabolism* by Brindley and Russel done on rats in which severe hardening of the arteries had been induced, and Redux prevented any further blood vessel damage!

The essential message of all these studies is that Redux can act synergistically with the weight loss it induces in order to alter an unfavorable biochemical process that may predispose you to cardiac disease and diabetes. It's impressive to note that these favorable biochemical changes usually did not require a long time to manifest; but often occurred within just a few short weeks. The exact mechanism by which Redux performs this Syndrome X "disappearing act" is not known at present. A great deal of research continues in this area. But the bottom line is that Redux has united cosmetic and medical weight loss. It works!

Just a Few Questions . . .

By approving Redux, the FDA has introduced some new questions, which need some answers. What makes Redux better than other "diet pills"? Does it resemble the amphetamines that used to be available for weight loss? Who should take Redux? How long should Redux be used? Can you take Redux for the rest of your life? All good questions, all to be answered shortly.

Until the 1970s, the only medications used for weight loss were amphetamines. Amphetamines have given somewhat of a tarnished reputation to weight-loss medications in general. It's not that amphetamines are terrible drugs in and of themselves, though they have side effects that include nervousness, inability to sleep, and palpitations, and are highly addictive. The real problem is that they can't be used for long periods of time, and many people abused them over time. And unfortunately, the illicit use of the drugs has made a bit of a comeback, targeting our youth. Amphetamines are currently used on the street, purportedly to give heightened sexual pleasure. While they are no longer used very much in weight loss, amphetamines are used to treat children who have the behavioral disorder known as attention deficit disorder (ADD), as well as those suffering from narcolepsy, a disorder that is characterized by the tendency to fall asleep without warning.

Interestingly, Redux and phen/fen (which we will discuss in Chapter 8) both have chemical structures similar to those of amphetamines. Many of you will read this and remember taking amphetamines in the past, and you may feel hesitant about taking Redux or phen/fen. However, there is no reason for concern. *Redux and phen/fen should not be confused with amphetamines. They are not amphetamines!*

So much for prescription weight-loss medications. Now what about other commonly available weight-loss aids? In its approval, the FDA said that Redux, which is a prescription drug, should be used only under a doctor's close supervision because of the risk of a rare pulmonary disorder. We will discuss this in greater detail in Chapter 4. Taking a regulated drug, such as Redux, requires that you go to a licensed medical doctor who will give you a written prescription for the drug, which must be filled at a pharmacy. Despite all the good results published in the studies of Redux, you may be thinking that you've heard similar claims for other "diet pills," which are less bothersome to take because they are available over the counter in drugstores or health food stores.

Let's take a moment to discuss the two most commonly used over-the-counter medications that are used for weight loss: chromium picolinate and phenylpropanolamine.

Chromium is a mineral normally found in the body in minute amounts. It functions to help insulin metabolize carbohydrates. Medicine has known about this function for decades. A study published in 1995 reported the effects of chromium picolinate on a group of college football players. It was found to increase their muscle mass and decrease their fat stores. Overnight, it seemed, the entire population started consuming large quantities of chromium picolinate. "New, improved" formulas emerged. Arnold Schwartzenegger must not have been too happy—after all those years of working out he learned that perhaps all he had really needed to muscle up was chromium picolinate! However, a subsequent and definitive study that was done at the University of Maryland

and appeared recently in the American College of Sports Medicine journal, *Medicine and Science in Sports and Exercise,* found chromium to be of no value in weight loss or putting on muscle. There won't be too many future studies on the relationship between chromium and weight loss; they aren't worth the money. If you are serious about weight loss, don't bother with this lightweight "miracle" weight-loss medication.

Phenylpropanolamine fares only slightly better. Contained in Dexatrim, phenylpropanolamine can cause slight weight loss—but it works better as a decongestant than as a weight-loss agent. It has been given to millions of patients by allergists and internists for chronic sinus problems, yet none of these people has reported a significant weight loss! Moreover, phenylpropanolamine was associated with so many bothersome side effects, such as tremors (the "shakes"), palpitations, and sleep disturbance, that it was ultimately withdrawn from the market for use as a decongestant.

Redux, by contrast, is a potent and serious medication for those who are serious about weight loss. If you fall into this category, you should first find out if you are a candidate for Redux (we'll discuss the restrictions in the next chapter). The FDA, in the guidelines it issued for the use of Redux, recommends the drug for anyone with a BMI over 30. If you don't know your BMI, go back to Chapter 1—it's easy to calculate. The example the FDA gives is someone who is 5'6" and over 186 pounds—that person would qualify for Redux. However, a patient with a BMI of 27 (for example, someone who was about the same height but weighed about 167 pounds) could also qualify if he or she had high blood pressure, diabetes, or any obesity-related medical disorder.

One of the FDA's concerns is that though Redux is well tolerated when prescribed for the right population, the drug will be overutilized and as a result we will see an increase in the incidence of side effects. Extrapolating from the FDA's guidelines for Redux, if your BMI is less than 25, you should not use Redux. That's clear enough; if your BMI is lower than 25, you probably don't need the kind of help that Redux offers. The problem is, what do we do with those people who have a BMI between 25 and 27 and have Syndrome X staring them in the face? Do we wait until symptoms of high blood pressure or diabetes appear? This is still a gray area. Ultimately, it will be a decision that you must make with your physician.

As for those of you who have five to ten pounds to lose: *You should not, in my opinion, take Redux.* Redux is a powerful drug that should be treated with respect, and for people with only a little weight to lose, the benefits don't outweigh the risks. But don't despair—*The Redux™ Revolution* can work for you without your taking the medication. You just need to follow the directions in the upcoming chapters.

The Road to Success

Redux is a new medication in this country, and chances are your doctor has never had firsthand experience with it. Therefore, it is very important that *you* understand how it works.

Your own Redux Revolution begins not when you take the pill, but when you change your attitude about weight loss based on the science we have reviewed. In fact, Redux is the technological outcome of the greatest weight-loss discovery of the century, which is the combination of what we have discovered about the obesity gene, leptin, neuropeptide Y, serotonin, and Redux. Without this wonderful antecedent research, Redux would not have been released.

The attitude change comes from the same source that we discussed earlier in this chapter—the upper part of the brain, which is associated with thinking and decision-making. This area is also associated with discipline. To establish your own success story, you must not be passive and assume that Redux will do all the work involved in weight loss. *This is not a passive program. You do not take Redux and then sit back, arms folded, and lose weight!*

The Redux™ Revolution requires that you take an active role from the outset. Even when you are taking Redux, the higher parts of the brain—those responsible for attitude, discipline, and decision-making—still control the hypothalamus and the appetite centers. They also modulate the effect of any weight-loss medication. Often when I ask patients how they feel they achieved their weight-loss goals, they respond that it was due to the weight-loss medication they received. This is a misconception, and I am always quick to point out that *they* lost the weight, *not* the medication. Their highest brain centers allowed them to use the medication correctly and obtain the best results from that medication. You lose weight with Redux's help, Redux does not lose weight for you.

However, the greatest gift Redux brings is that it takes the place of willpower, which from time immemorial has been the basis of all diets. There is no longer a need to take a deep breath and say, "Willpower? Here we go again," because willpower has never, ever lasted long enough for you to keep the weight off.

The Redux™ Revolution will help you stop yo-yoing once and for all. With Redux, you take a small white capsule, and in doing so, you are affirming your commitment to assuming the all-important new attitude. You will suffer neither the physical pains of hunger nor the psychological stress of being on a diet.

Redux works within one hour. Redux doesn't elevate metabolism or burn fat. Redux's action on the brain is imperceptible, so you don't really feel anything at all. Most people describe feeling good, whether because of the mood elevation that comes from more serotonin in the hypothalamus or because of the knowledge that they have finally taken action to do something about their weight that does not involve so much self-sacrifice.

The first time you eat after starting Redux, you will notice that you won't eat as much. Perhaps you will feel full sooner, after having eaten less food. In between this meal and the next, you should not feel hungry. Even if you do not experience this best-case scenario, that's fine: Redux will still diminish your appetite and between-meal cravings to some extent. Again, Redux does not work for everyone, but its track record is undeniable. This process continues every day. Weight loss is based on your diminished daily caloric intake while maintaining the same level of activity.

Soon you begin to interface with Redux's most powerful positive side effect—*it has the ability to end the preoccupation with food that most overweight people experience.* This preoccupation with food is manifested by constant thoughts of food, especially between meals. No sooner do you finish breakfast than you're entertaining options for lunch. You eat lunch and think, "What's for dinner?" At dinner you wonder what to snack on later. And so it goes. This also sets the stage for eventual bingeing and emotional eating.

All these thoughts of food occupy a large percent of your daily thought capacity, hampering you in your pursuit of your everyday routines. Because it shuts down the appetite center,

Redux can end this abnormal thought content. Redux can also end the constant worry about each individual food choice: Is this food "good" or "bad"? Redux takes away the power that we have attributed to food and returns it to us. This phenomenon was described best to me by M.C., an overweight school administrator. When taking fenfluramine (Redux's sister drug), she told me that "the food cabinets in the kitchen no longer call me." In fact, during a period when she had run out of the pills, she said that she heard the cabinets "calling again." Incidentally, she has lost 50 pounds and looks marvelous!

As you lose weight taking Redux, your attitude will probably change. You will realize that this new science really does put you back in sync with your own body. You really do lose weight with Redux, without walking around feeling hungry and constantly thinking about food. Now come new questions:

- How much can I lose in one month? How much in six?
- How long can I take Redux?
- Does Redux interfere with other medications I take?
- What should I eat while taking Redux?
- What about exercise?

All of these questions, and more, will soon be answered. The answers may surprise you!

DID YOU KNOW . . .

- Redux has been used by millions worldwide for more than ten years.
- The word "placebo" means "I shall please" in Latin.

• Some patients enrolled in studies actually become addicted to the placebo.

• Foods that contain serotonin include bananas, avocados, walnuts, plums, and pineapples.

• Medications that cause weight loss are called anorexigens.

Chapter 4

Redux: Safety, Side Effects, and Risks

In Chapter 3, we discussed the fact that with the Redux Revolution, you're in control. Part of being in control involves learning all you can about the pros and cons of taking Redux. We have already talked about how Redux works in the brain. Now let's look at the safety issues you should be aware of when deciding whether or not to use Redux.

Safety is a natural human preoccupation. We're all concerned about safe neighborhoods, safe drinking water, and safe products for ourselves and our children. The concern for safety is particularly strong when the subject is drugs. We want to make sure that anything we put inside our bodies will, at the very least, do us no harm.

Since Redux received FDA approval, we know that it was scrutinized by the medical and scientific communities and was deemed to be safe. However, Redux is a drug, and like all drugs, it carries some risks to users. There have been a number of sensationalized reports in the media about the possible dangers of this drug. How serious are these dangers? To put this matter into perspective, let's take a look at a few other medications, used by millions of people, that are generally considered beyond reproach.

Beyond Reproach?

Each day, tens of thousands of asthmatic American children receive a painful injection that has potentially lethal consequences and has killed in the past. This injection has been viewed by some as so dangerous that its use has been abandoned in the United Kingdom. Possible side effects of this medication include life-threatening asthma and choking. What is even more surprising is that these injections do not work any better than readily available safe alternatives. That's assuming they work at all! So, what is this drug that we push into children's arms even though England has said "no way" to it? Allergy shots!

Allergy shots are by no means alone in their potential for danger. There are many other common medications that we take, without much thought, that may cause harm. In fact, each day hundreds of thousands of people take two medications that have caused severe, life-threatening reactions and deaths: aspirin and penicillin. Yet no exposé has been done on these billion-dollar mainstays of the drug industry. Why? Because public perception says that they are safe; and despite these recognized side effects, they are!

All drugs—anti-inflammatories, antibiotics, antihypertensives, and weight-loss drugs such as Redux—have side effects. Even over-the-counter medications have side effects, which may include drowsiness, insomnia, stomach pain, diarrhea, and headache. As we will see, these common ailments are also possible side effects of Redux. Again, all drugs have side effects. In order to make an evaluation for safety, each medication's side-effects profile must be evaluated by itself, compared to those of other drugs within its class, and compared to those of medications outside its class. Only then will we have the proper side-effect perspective—and "perspective" is the key word here.

No sooner had Redux been approved by the FDA than some elements of the popular media brought into tight focus—and paid almost exclusive attention to—the drug's most serious side effects. Arresting sound bites such as "This drug causes brain damage" and "This drug causes irreversible lung problems" soon flooded the airwaves. But anyone wanting to focus attention on a medication that has brain damage and lung problems as listed side effects would not need to point to a new drug such as Redux. In fact, brain damage and lung problems are known side effects of ibuprofen, a common painkiller that is available over the counter! While rare, these side effects do occur, and yet they seldom deter anyone from taking ibuprofen—nor should they. These severe, sometimes fatal, side effects occur in such small numbers that few users of ibuprofen even take them into consideration when looking to ease the pain of headaches and arthritis. Theoretically, the side-effect risks increase over time and with increased use of the drug; therefore, the more you use ibuprofen, the higher your risk. Still, this information will hardly affect the use of one of the most popular drugs in history. This is because the overall reputation of ibuprofen—the perspective we have on it—tells us that it's safe, and unless there is an outbreak of unexpected side effects, ibuprofen will remain popular. Again, it is all a matter of side-effect perspective.

Side Effects: What You Need to Know

Ultimately, it will be you and your doctor who decide whether you should take Redux. Therefore, you will have to form your own perspective on side effects. This chapter is intended to help you do just that. It will give you a detailed look at the possible side effects of Redux.

When the FDA made its decision to approve Redux, its number-one priority was to ensure that the drug is safe. The material the FDA reviewed to make this determination is the basis for the following Redux safety profile. Keep in mind that Redux has been used by an estimated 10 million people, worldwide, over the last ten years. That amounts to millions upon millions of doses consumed, without any major side effects on a large scale.

One of the first concerns about any medication is the issue of control. With Redux, this is not a problem. Although Redux interacts with parts of the brain and can affect mood, it is not addictive, either physically or psychologically. Redux does not "take over your body"; it does not control you. As we discussed in the previous chapter, you are always in control because it is your cerebral cortex—the active, deciding, reasoning part of the brain—that, in large measure, controls the way you eat and use Redux.

But while control is not the problem with Redux, there are several side effects.

In general, drug side effects can be divided into two categories, short-term and long-term. Short-term side effects do not last a long time and cease when the drug is stopped; they are usually not severe. Long-term side effects may continue after the drug is stopped; they are due to an accumulation of the drug in a particular organ, which causes a toxic reaction in the organ. For example, alcohol in excessive amounts is toxic to the liver, and the chemotherapy agent adriamycin accumulates in the heart muscle and can damage it and cause heart failure.

Most of Redux's side effects fall into the first category—short-term. This is because, in humans, the drug does not accumulate in any organ. However, there have been scattered reports that the drug causes one long-range and serious medical problem. We will examine this in further detail later in this chapter. First, we will examine the most common side effects, which are likely to be experienced by many users.

Dry Mouth

Dry mouth is the most common side effect of Redux. It is manifested by a slight "cotton-mouth" feeling, with patients usually feeling the need to moisten their lips. Any medication that works on the central nervous system, such as antidepressant and anti-anxiety medications, can have the same effect, as can antihistamines. This side effect is a nuisance but has no other implication. It can sometimes disappear by itself, or increased water intake may alleviate the discomfort. Patients rarely discontinue the medication because of this side effect.

Can You Stomach Redux?

Some of Redux's more common side effects are manifested in the gastrointestinal tract: the stomach and the intestines. This phenomenon is probably due to the fact that these parts of the body have cells that contain serotonin. Even though serotonin is a neurotransmitter usually associated with the brain, it is also found in many other parts of the body. Gastrointestinal side effects of Redux can range from abdominal pain to nausea. The most common side effect is diarrhea. Of the 1,159 patients in the 17 Redux studies analyzed and presented to the FDA by Interneuron, about 200 reported having diarrhea, which apparently was mild, because it did not lead to discontinuation of the drug. Patients were able to continue Redux because the diarrhea stopped on its own, without any intervention. Relatively uncommon is a mild, non-crampy abdominal pain that can come and go. Rarely, a patient reported experiencing nausea and/or vomiting.

To put these symptoms into side-effect perspective, all of these abdominal symptoms are far more common in patients who take the group of medications called nonsteroidal anti-inflammatory drugs (NSAIDs). These include aspirin, ibuprofen, and naproxen, commonly used for arthritis inflammation and pain. Many of you have taken these medications, despite the side effects listed above. There is one very major difference between this group of medications and Redux, though. NSAIDs can also lead to erosions in the stomach and to severe gastric bleeding episodes, some of which have been fatal. Redux is not associated with any of these serious side effects. Which is safer, then—aspirin or Redux? You decide. It's all a matter of perspective!

Too Tired?

Drowsiness can be a side effect of Redux. It can range from mild lethargy to overt sleepiness. It is recommended that a patient not drive or operate any potentially dangerous machinery when taking the first doses of Redux. Over time, this feeling of drowsiness may disappear by itself; it may never appear in the first place. Some patients stop the medication because of this side effect.

The Cerebral Type

Some of Redux's side effects are due to its causing serotonin to accumulate in a tiny area of the hypothalamus, leaving another area relatively devoid of serotonin. This is called "pooling." When the areas of the hypothalamus that affect sleep, moods, and memory are affected, the symptoms will reflect the specific area that is deficient in serotonin. All of these symptoms are reversible upon stopping the medication. They include:

Depression. This side effect is more prevalent with the use of Redux's sister drug, fenfluramine (Pondimin). Since depression is relatively uncommon with the use of Pondimin, it is considered a rare side effect in Redux. All drugs that involve high levels of serotonin can cause depression including Prozac and Zoloft—which are, ironically, antidepressants! The depression that may result from the use of Redux is not a profound type, and ranges from a certain "unworldly" feeling to losing interest in everyday activities. There is no residual depression when the drug is stopped. Clinicians should be aware that many overweight patients suffer from depression, so Redux may simply unmask a subclinical depression. In my opinion, any patient who exhibits depression while on Redux should be further evaluated for depression.

Anxiety. The anxiety that may be caused by Redux should not be compared with the kind associated with amphetamines—it is far less intense. The descriptions I most often hear of this anxiety are being nervous, feeling "antsy," feeling unable to sit still, and needing to repeat an activity constantly, like cleaning the house. This anxiety, too, goes away when the drug is discontinued.

Sleep disturbances. These occur in users of Redux on occasion and can range from having difficulty falling asleep to sleeping too much. Some people have dream disturbances as well. These range from unusually vivid dreams to outright nightmares.

Headache. Redux can cause headache, as can just about all medications. In fact, migraine headache medications can actually cause headaches to get worse rather than better. Often the headaches disappear in four to eight hours.

Memory loss. This side effect caught the public's attention because of reports relating to fenfluramine (Pondimin). Perhaps concerns are high in this area because the public perceives this condition to be a precursor to Alzheimer's disease. However, the memory loss involved with Redux is transitory—it is not long-lasting and involves only short-term memory. Common examples include forgetting keys, a phone number, or an appointment. The memory loss reverses upon discontinuation of the drug and has nothing to do with Alzheimer's disease.

All of these side effects are more than just nuisances and have caused some patients to stop taking the medication. However, many of these side effects do become tolerable over time.

The following case history will illustrate the tolerability of the bulk of the side effects we just reviewed. R.S. is a single 40-year-old woman. She had come into my office somewhat reluctantly. Having failed at weight loss many times before, she was not expecting much in the way of results. I started her on Redux. She called back three days later saying that she couldn't sleep. I told her to take the drug earlier in the day. Two days later, I received another phone call—the sleep disturbance was gone, but now she was feeling "spacey." She said nothing about her appetite being suppressed. Four days later, she called again. This time it was slight nausea. I suggested that she stop the medication and that we try a different one on her next visit. "Are you kidding?" she asked. "I feel great and I already lost six pounds."

R.S.'s situation is very unusual, since it's a rare patient indeed who experiences more than one side effect, let alone several sequentially. But what's interesting is that even though she did experience side effects, their effect was transient and mild and in no real way disturbed her quality of life, and she wanted to stay on the drug.

This has been a common experience. Sometimes patients call for reassurance that the minor side effects are due to the drug and not their weight loss. Often they are so buoyed by their success that the side effects tend to be tolerated, and eventually they vanish. However, there is a certain percentage of patients who will not be able to tolerate Redux and who will have to be switched to a different medication. It seems that most of the side effects we have reviewed develop early and can be corrected by changing the dose or by changing the timing of the dose. Again, these concerns should be addressed with your doctor both before you take Redux and while you're taking it.

Some Nerve

You may have heard that Redux causes nerve damage. This has been seen in a small number of studies of monkeys, one of them done at Johns Hopkins University. Redux has not been found to cause nerve damage in humans. The study upon which the original observation was based, entitled "Dexfenfluramine Neurotoxicity in the Brains of Nonhuman Primates," appeared in *Lancet* in 1991. The monkeys received doses that were much higher than the human dose. The FDA, on reviewing the data, found that this nerve damage has been seen only in animals so far. Again, the ultimate choice is yours, but this side effect has never been seen in humans. In addition, a follow-up study in mice refuted the original study.

Drug Interactions

Although Redux has few adverse interactions with other medications, it should be used with caution when taken with any other drugs that affect the central nervous system, such as antidepressants, anti-anxiety medications, and sleeping pills. You should not have general anesthesia with Redux in your system. Also, in my opinion, you should not take Redux with certain blood pressure pills. Moreover, a rare constellation of symptoms known as the "serotonin syndrome" has been reported when using medications that involve the serotonin system along with Redux. These medications include anti-migraine agents and antidepressives. For more information, see Chapter 13, question #1. Do not use Redux with another weight-loss medication. All of these possible drug interactions should be discussed with your doctor.

Remember, always consult your physician if you have any questions about dosage, side effects, or possible drug interactions. Most of the side effects associated with Redux are dose-dependent. This means that the more medication you take, the more side effects you are likely to have. Therefore, always take the smallest dose of Redux possible!

Contraindications

Contraindications are situations where use of the drug is prohibited. Pregnant or nursing women should not take Redux. In my opinion, patients with severe high blood pressure, heart disease, or glaucoma should also avoid the drug. Although no studies have been done in this area, caution should be exercised in giving the drug to patients with kidney or liver disease. And although drug abuse potential is low, Redux should not be given to alcohol or drug abusers. The drug should not be administered under any circumstances to patients diagnosed with primary pulmonary hypertension (PPH; see below), patients taking monoamine oxidase (MAO) inhibitors, or patients who are allergic to dexfenfluramine, fenfluramine, and related compounds.

PPH—A Serious Risk?

So far we have been talking about side effects that are usually reversible. However, there is one Redux side effect that has gotten a great deal of media attention and can have life-

77

threatening implications. It is called primary pulmonary hypertension (PPH), and a warning for it appears on the Redux package insert. This is not to be confused with hypertension, which is another word for high blood pressure, or with pulmonary hypertension that occurs in the wake of another disease.

Primary pulmonary hypertension occurs when the blood vessels that carry blood from the heart to the lungs become narrowed. This causes pressure to back up to the heart and can induce heart failure. Treatment is available in the form of medications, but a heart-lung transplant may be necessary if medication is unsuccessful. PPH has caused fatalities. Unfortunately, there is no blood test or X ray to diagnose PPH before you fully contract it. It can sometimes spontaneously reverse itself with discontinued use of the weight-loss drug. Symptoms include chest pain, shortness of breath on exertion, fainting, and edema (water retention) in the legs and feet.

Should any of these symptoms occur, the patient should stop taking the weight-loss drug immediately and notify the doctor. This warning is of utmost importance because PPH can often reverse itself spontaneously upon discontinuation of the weight-loss drug.

This condition is extremely rare, occurring in an estimated one in 40,000 patients on Redux. To put this into side-effect perspective, fenfluramine (Pondimin), the "sister" to Redux, is also associated with PPH. This FDA-approved drug has been used for more than 25 years in Europe and the United States. In that time, according to the manufacturer's label, it has caused only four cases of PPH. Two cases reversed themselves when the drug was stopped, one responded to medical treatment, and one case was fatal. The FDA took these cases, as well as the cases from Europe, into consideration when Redux was approved, and felt that the drug's benefits far outweighed its risks. Still, however small the possibility of acquiring PPH, you and your physician must take this side effect into consideration when deciding whether or not you should take Redux. Here are a few precepts to help you guard against PPH:

• The FDA's prescribing guidelines for Redux should be respected. Redux should not be used by thin people trying to get thinner! Following the FDA's guidelines will lower the number of patients at risk for the disease. If your BMI is too low for you to qualify for Redux, and you still want to lose weight, the weight-loss plan described later in *The Redux™ Revolution* will work for you—without your needing to take Redux!

• Consider taking "drug holidays" when on Redux. PPH is not a condition that you get on the first, the second, or even the twentieth dose. In all likelihood, it probably takes several months, or longer, of taking the drug before PPH is manifested. The use of "drug holidays"—when you stop taking the drug periodically—could be beneficial in this respect. This idea will be covered in detail in Chapter 7. Of course, using the lowest dose of Redux possible is still of utmost importance. However, there is a possibility that with further research on PPH and Redux, it will be found that there is an idiosyncratic relationship between the two, meaning that any amount of Redux can cause PPH. This concern will be addressed in upcoming studies.

• Stop taking Redux if it isn't really working for you. According to Redux's manufacturer, only those who lose four pounds during the first month on Redux will go on to lose any significant weight in the ensuing year. Should you not achieve this modest goal, I suggest you stop taking Redux after one month and switch to another medication.

• PPH is rare, but by far more commonly seen in individuals who are not taking Redux or any other drugs. PPH is so rare that many a pulmonary specialist has never seen a case of it. In the general population, PPH is estimated to occur in one or two people per million per year. Interestingly, people with a Body Mass Index above 30 have a twofold increase in risk of developing PPH. As of this writing, there has been no study that directly implicates Redux or Pondimin as the cause of PPH. However, for those who are taking Redux, it is estimated that the number of cases of PPH will rise to 18 cases per million per year.

• PPH is five times more common in women than men, and the median age for those who have PPH is 35. This profile is very similar to the demographics of women who diet in general. The association between Redux (and other weight-loss medications) and PPH may be coincidental. In any event, more studies are needed to establish a cause-and-effect relationship between Redux and PPH.

Talk to your doctor about PPH before starting Redux. You must be totally comfortable with your choice of whether Redux is for you. Try not to get caught up in the sensationalism that accompanies a new drug's release. You can always wait and take Redux at a later time, if you so choose.

I hope you take Redux's side-effect profile into consideration before you decide to take it. Because any newly released drug is closely followed in post-market evaluations, your doctor would be able to notify you immediately should any additional side effects or problems be discovered. And finally, to put Redux's most feared complication—PPH—into perspective, consider this: England, which has a very conservative medical establishment, has deemed Redux safe to use for three months at a time, and yet it has abandoned allergy shots for asthma because they are considered too dangerous.

Now that you've got some side-effect perspective, it's time to take the next step in the Redux Revolution. The next two chapters will reveal the role that diet and exercise can play in maximizing your weight loss, whether or not you and your doctor decide that Redux is right for you.

DID YOU KNOW . . .

• Approximately 5% of all hospital admissions are due to adverse drug reactions or side effects, such as having low potassium levels from diuretics, a potentially life-threatening situation.

• 10% to 20% of all hospital patients experience side effects from medications.

• The most common cause of death from medication is bleeding from the gastrointestinal tract, which is caused by aspirin and related drugs.

• One-third to one-half of all patients make errors when taking medications.

• Drug allergies can cause adverse drug reactions, but are rarely fatal.

• The most common adverse drug reaction is a skin rash.

Chapter 5

Redux and Your Diet

If you and your doctor have evaluated Redux's side-effect profile, discussed your medical history, and decided that you are a candidate for Redux, you need a plan that you can follow easily—a plan that you can live with. Providing this plan is the main goal of the next three chapters. They should be read together. Remember, Redux is not to be thought of as a crutch or as a "last resort" for those of you who may have given up in your quest to be thinner. *Redux is a tool that can provide the impetus you need to establish minimal lifestyle changes leading to permanent weight loss.* Toward this end, *The Redux™ Revolution* utilizes the best diet in the world, the diet that has kept you thriving all these years: *your diet!*

Each of us has unique food preferences, unlike anyone else's on the planet! This is our gastronomic fingerprint, and it's part of what makes each of us special. Imagine for a moment that you were wrongly convicted of a capital crime and tonight you will be served your last meal. What would you pick? Would it be a prepackaged commercial diet-plan meal? Would it be a boring salad and bland low-fat chicken? I doubt it! You would choose the same high-fat, high-carbohydrate food that you have been craving since your basic food preferences were established—at about age two! These are the same foods you will crave for the rest of your days.

By now, all of you know what healthy eating is and what it is not. Chances are, your diet contains many healthy choices as well as some that are not so healthy. In my opinion, Redux will serve you best by allowing you to lose weight while eating the foods you like—just in smaller quantities!

You will lose weight with your own diet. While you won't be able to continue eating 15 slices of bread a day, a quart of ice cream, or a pound of cheese, Redux will lessen the amount of food you ingest—no matter how "unhealthy" your diet. In this fashion, you will be able to eat ice cream, cake, even cookies; you will just be eating smaller amounts of them. Dieting, as we know it, puts far too much pressure on you. With conventional diets, not only must you decrease your total caloric intake, but you are forced to change your entire eating lifestyle. You're limited to low-fat (high-protein, high-carbohydrate) foods, salads, four to eight servings of fruit a day, and grains. Ice cream, cake, and cookies are out of the question! The premise behind these plans is to get you to lose weight and develop healthy eating habits at the same time. I believe this goal is too difficult and sets the dieter up for eventual failure. Redux can provide a simpler, more natural sequence. By inhibiting your appetite, Redux enables you to lose weight. While you lose weight, you learn what eating habits and food choices work for you.

As I tell my patients, the whole idea behind appetite suppressants is to allow you to see how much food you can eat and still lose weight. I provide my patients with a weight-loss framework based on the use of appetite suppressants, allowing them to plug in their individual food choices. A comprehensive plan is necessary, because at some point you must finally stop taking the medication and rely on your own habits and choices. You not only need to know how to use Redux, you need to create a plan for the post-medication period, and you need to practice it while you're on the medication. I don't tell patients what to eat; I show them *how* to eat, without dictating food choices. Of course, there are people out there who still want to continue on their favorite "diet" or a commercial diet plan. They can still use Redux. Redux will work with almost any diet plan, provided you follow the directions outlined in this chapter and the one that follows.

Studies have shown that Redux works when used in conjunction with various 1,400-to-1,500-calorie diets. No difference in weight loss was seen in patients following high-protein, low-fat, or low-carbohydrate diets. These diets are called macronutrient diets. The current macronutrient diet of choice is a low-fat diet. Yet, did you know that in the past decade, our fat intake has *decreased* while our average weights have actually *increased*? This is happening because we have been duped into thinking that low-fat foods would be the answer to our weight-loss problems. We are getting heavier and heavier on low-fat foods! If *The Redux™ Revolution* is to be the fresh approach you are looking for, it's time to stop the diet-cult macronutrient approach. It is important to note that when Redux was tested with a low-calorie diet (under 800 calories per day), it didn't work as well. Very-low-calorie diets should not be used when taking Redux—you must eat!

While Redux is the star of this book, the star of your weight loss is *you*. Redux assists you in making the important lifestyle changes that you are about to learn. Our goal is to have this process occur in an orderly fashion; the body demands order, not chaos. Let's begin by solving one of the body's mysteries: How rapidly do our bodies let us lose fat? Two important studies, one done recently and the other conducted during World War II, will answer this important question for us.

Not So Fast!

In a study recently published in the *New England Journal of Medicine,* researchers put a group of overweight people on an 800-calorie-a-day liquid diet. During this study, their leptin levels were measured. Incredibly, after only a 10% drop in body fat, leptin levels dropped over 50%! Remember, when leptin levels fall, the neuropeptide Y in our brain increases our appetite, and we regain any weight lost. This disproportionate drop in leptin indicates that the brain is extremely vigilant in detecting initial weight loss. If you lose weight too quickly, alarms go off in the brain. An increase in neuropeptide Y increases appetite. This explains why if you are obese, "quickie" weight-loss regimens of any kind must always fail. You are literally telling your brain to increase your appetite. This message, though, can be blunted by Redux. Now, let's look at the second study.

Soldiers' Story

Early in World War II, the U.S. government conducted a study on starvation using young, healthy military volunteers. They were essentially semistarved for six months! During this period, some took in slightly more calories than others.

Fat and lean body mass were measured over time. During the first five days, *no fat* was lost at all, only muscle and water. After one week of semistarvation, only one to two pounds of fat were lost. After that, the weight-loss rate was about two pounds per week. Fat continued to be lost, as did muscle, until about the two-to-three-month mark. After this point, *no further weight was lost.* Surprisingly, the metabolic rates of the soldiers went down by about 33%. Their bodies were literally fighting against further weight loss.

We owe a great debt to these brave men. They teach us that no matter what kind of diet you try—high-carbohydrate, low-fat, high-protein, low-carbohydrate—and no matter how many calories you ingest, your body can lose only a certain amount of fat, and it does so at a predetermined rate. If you lose too much weight too quickly, it will cause an increase in neuropeptide Y, as well as a decrease in your metabolism. Both of these factors cause an increase in hunger and lead to weight gain. The only way out of this dilemma is to lose weight in an orderly, slow fashion, so as to lull the brain into thinking no weight loss is occurring. This method also ensures that you won't lose too much muscle. We want to sneak those first few pounds off! Imagine a dishonest bank teller at her first day of work. She pockets $10,000. All the alarms go off, and she is handcuffed and led to the squad car. Now, imagine that the same teller instead pockets 50 cents here, a dollar there. By the time she is caught . . . well, you understand.

The single most important "weight-loss tip" of this new science is: *To be successful at weight loss, the first few pounds must come off at a slow, steady rate.* This is the exact opposite of what we are accustomed to hearing! What is the best rate for you to lose weight? The all-important answer comes from these two studies. Ideally, you should strive to lose *about 1% of your total initial body weight per week.* The easiest way to come up with your personal weekly weight-loss target is to take your body weight, and place a decimal point two digits from the right. For example, if you weigh 225 pounds, you should strive to lose 2.25 pounds per week. If you weigh 170 pounds, your weekly weight-loss target would be 1.7 pounds per week.

One pound of fat is essentially the size and weight of a softball. Shedding two and a half softballs off your body in one week is a marvelous accomplishment! If you try to exceed this rate, you will trip two of the brain's "fail-safe" mechanisms, one short-term, the other long term. The short term mechanism guards against large amounts of weight loss by increasing neuropeptide Y, which raises your appetite and lowers your metabolic rate. We will soon take a closer look at metabolism, but for right now think of it as body heat. The soldiers' experience taught us that in losing weight through starvation, you lose only muscle and water the first few days. Muscle is a metabolically active tissue that burns calories 24 hours a day and creates heat. By losing this valuable muscle tissue, which is not easily replaced in women, you lose a major source of heat production. The body's thermostat in the hypothalamus tries to counter this by instructing the body to store fat (fat is a potential depot for future heat production), or by increasing appetite (which will provide fuel to raise the body heat, a.k.a. metabolism). If you continue to stress this short-term mechanism by continued calorie restriction, you trip the body's set point, which is also located in the hypothalamus. The set point guards against long-term change in weight. It does this by alerting the metabolism to burn calories more slowly. This is why a slow initial rate of fat loss is crucial in setting up future *permanent* fat loss. You will not reach your goals by rushing and stressing your body.

How long should this organized rate of fat loss continue? By my estimation, you should adopt this slow and steady approach until your weight loss reaches approximately 5% of your initial body weight. This figure is based on the results of the first study I cited, where 10% fat loss meant 50% decrease in leptin and a theoretical increase in appetite. For this reason, we don't want to get to the 10% mark too quickly. Here is an example. A woman weighs 180 pounds. She wants to know what her rate of weight loss should be so as to keep her brain's "fail-safe" mechanisms inactive. Place a decimal point after the first digit in her weight. That gives us a target weight loss of 1.8 pounds per week, and 5% of her initial body weight would be nine pounds. This means that she should pace herself so that she takes slightly more than four weeks (9 ÷ 1.8) to reach this nine-pound goal. Keep in mind that these figures are approximate and represent the "best-case scenario." One percent of your total initial body weight per week, up to approximately 5% of your initial body weight, is the rate, as well as the limit, of body-fat loss that you should attempt to achieve in order to keep your brain from sabotaging your weight-loss effort. Losing less than 1% of body weight per week is fine; just keep in mind that losing at least four pounds in the first month is crucial in order for Redux to be effective in the long run. This "rate-of-weight-loss" concept is my own and is based on my experience with more than 2,000 patients.

The Body Rules

Before you take Redux for the first time, it is important that you remember the Body Rules we have just learned. The basic concept is to keep your metabolism as high as possible, from day one of your weight-loss effort. Here's a summary:

- Respect your body—don't starve it. *You must eat if Redux is to work.* If you don't, you will only lose valuable calorie-burning muscle.
- Each of us has a special rate of fat loss. The initial rate of weight loss is crucial for long-term success. Calculate your ideal initial rate of weight loss as shown earlier in this chapter and do not try to exceed it. If you do, you will once again lose muscle and trip the body's weight-gain mechanisms.

By following these two Body Rules, you lower your level of leptin slowly. In doing this, you are not only tricking the brain into thinking that no weight is being lost, but, like the twins I mentioned in Chapter 2, you may actually be fooling the obesity gene. After this initial weight loss is accomplished, you can proceed at any rate you wish—provided you follow the rest of the program outlined in this book.

There is another reason to proceed slowly. In Chapter 2 we were introduced to the concept of hyperinsulinemia. The obese have high levels of insulin, which can drive their hunger. If you lose weight too quickly, you will stress the body and insulin levels will ultimately rise even higher. You will be hungrier than before—and even heavier!

With all of these terrific reasons why a person should not lose weight too quickly, I offer no apologies to those who "must lose 30 pounds by Monday." This attitude sets people up for failure. Remember, weight loss is a lifelong endeavor! Redux will make the entire weight-loss process easier, so that you aren't struggling to lose those initial few pounds. Best of all, *The Redux*™ *Revolution* will now show you a way of fine-tuning your food intake so that you can work with Redux and lose weight by using *your diet, not mine.*

Your Diet, Not Mine!

There are only three major nutrients that constitute all of our food: fat, carbohydrates, and protein. Protein plays no role in weight gain or weight loss. This is due to two factors:

First, protein is not stored by the body. It is used in the construction and replacement of worn-out proteins. Since protein does not accumulate in the body, any excess protein is changed into carbohydrate. This process uses up energy, but because the amount of calories burned to do this is so small, it has no effect on weight loss.

Second, humans eat very little protein, in general. While we do need it to survive, we don't need much. Even if you were to follow the pro-protein gurus, you would still only be eating 75–100 grams of protein a day. This is only about 300–400 calories per day. Most of us eat about 35–50 grams of protein (or roughly 140–200 protein calories) each day. This is based on the fact that one gram of protein equals four calories, the same as for carbohydrates.

Moreover, of all the macronutrient dieting techniques, the one that involves adding protein to the diet is the one most fraught with problems. It is extremely hard and tedious to follow. Also, many protein sources, such as meats and cheeses, have considerable fat content. When you follow a high-protein diet, you are essentially adding fat calories to your diet for no reason.

Research has established that fats are the main dietary culprits that help cause and sustain our being overweight. Scientists tell us that we love the taste of fat, and the heavier you are, the more you crave it! Fats contain nine calories per gram, more than double the calorie count of carbohydrates (sugars). Butter, lard, and the fatty content of steak are examples of "solitary" fats. However, few people eat fat by itself.

A quick list of the top five foods that overweight men and women consume demonstrates that few people like fats by themselves. They like their fats with carbohydrates! In essence, the carbohydrates just go along for a ride with the fats, but together, sugar and fat are a hard-to-beat taste combination. Redux can play a big role in appetite control because it specifically inhibits our appetite for carbohydrates and, indirectly, fats. The lists below are not "snack lists," but lists of the staple foods preferred, based on my patient surveys.

WOMEN	MEN
1. Bread, crackers, rolls	1. Bread, crackers, rolls
2. Cookies, cakes	2. Ice cream
3. Ice cream, yogurt	3. Cookies, cakes
4. Meats	4. Meats
5. Pasta	5. Poultry

For women and men, the "top three" are foods loaded with fats and carbohydrates! Somehow, the snacks of childhood have evolved into the food staples of adults. Redux can lower your desire for these foods, make you eat less of these foods, and make you feel more satisfied eating smaller quantities. The reason for this is that the higher the levels of serotonin in the hypothalamus (which are raised by Redux), the lower our desire for carbohydrates. This indirectly lowers the amount of fat we take in. As we move down the lists, the choices become healthier and "less fattening"—like meats, poultry, and pasta. How do we know that you will choose the healthier foods and not choose the cakes, cookies, and ice cream? We don't! But we don't really care at first, remember, so long as weight is lost slowly. Redux preferentially lowers the desire for carbohydrates and fats—the ingredients of all binges. Since we don't get heavy by eating too much protein—red meat, fish, and chicken—Redux will effectively lower your calorie intake and cause weight loss, even if you insist on some of the high-fat/high-carbohydrate choices on the lists. As you lose weight, you will be able to practice eating healthier foods at your own pace. We take a closer look at developing new eating habits in Chapter 7, "Life After Redux." However, to summarize *The Redux™ Revolution*'s preferred macronutrient eating strategy, it is moderate fat intake and moderate carbohydrate intake.

If you follow the Body Rules we outlined previously, you will still be taking in a fair amount of food, no matter what you choose to eat. Redux best serves you not simply by suppressing your appetite but by altering it. It eliminates the preoccupation with food that so many overweight people experience. You won't crave the foods you used to. This lack of craving will allow you to make smarter food choices without the undue pressure of intense caloric restriction and the constant necessity of making healthy food choices that often accompanies conventional diets. However, you can help Redux along by remembering that each of us has a key weight-gain food. This is the food that we know we like, that tastes great, and that usually causes our downfall when we're on a diet. For me, it was peanut butter—and I haven't touched it in two years. Identify your key food and keep away from it, with the help of Redux, of course. Some key foods that patients often mistake for healthy choices include hard cheeses, nuts, cold cuts, and peanut butter. Hard cheeses include Swiss, American, provolone, and Muenster, among others. Soft white cheeses, like farmer's cheese, cottage cheese, and pot cheese, are better choices. Key weight-gain foods have a common denominator—an inordinate percentage of their total calories are fat calories. While many of them do contain protein, they do not contain enough to justify their over-consumption. Also, fried foods of any kind should be eaten in modest quantities only—perhaps only on weekends.

Another suggestion I would make is to choose to eliminate 200 to 300 calories per day from your diet. Weight loss requires some caloric restriction, and Redux accomplishes this by suppressing your appetite. A small additional caloric reduction such as the one I'm suggesting is a way to augment the calorie-restriction process begun by Redux. This doesn't mean you must forgo your favorite foods. A calorie is a calorie, to your body. The body's weight-loss mechanisms do not care which foods are eliminated to reach this suggested reduction. It's your choice—you are in control!

Keep in mind, these are only suggestions! As long as you respect the Body Rules, weight loss will follow! It really is that simple! In the short run, you will lose weight, but it's important to learn to change your way of eating for the future, when you stop Redux. We also stated previously that *The Redux™ Revolution* is an active plan, not a passive pill-taking plan. If there is ever a time to learn how to eat healthfully, it is *now*. Redux gives you this opportunity by taking away the pressure of having to make "perfect" eating choices every time. As I tell my patients who are on phen/fen, and now Redux, *The Redux™ Revolution* is not about counting calories. However, you should know the caloric counts of the foods on the "top five" list. Your body counts calories because our brains have thermic, or heat, sensors that measure the amount of heat developed in the body at any given time. The food we eat contains calories, and we need a minimal amount of calories to keep these thermal sensors from being alerted and tampering with our metabolic rate. All you are asked to do here is work with your body and *delete the 200 to 300 calories daily* by exercising some portion control, with the help of Redux. This conscious cutting back of calories, as opposed to letting Redux do all the work (though it does most of the work), is the key to long-term weight loss, as we will see in Chapter 7.

Say "NOEP"—The National Overweight Eating Pattern

Overweight people tend to fight their own metabolisms. Here's why. There exists what I call the national overweight eating pattern. This is the eating pattern of 95% of my patients. After having a big, late dinner, and then late-night snacks, they rarely wake up hungry. If they do decide to eat breakfast, they eat what I call the national overweight breakfast—bagels and cream cheese or a plain bagel. Many just skip breakfast. In fact, many of my patients tell me that if they've eaten breakfast, they've "blown the whole day." This means that they can justify eating whatever they want to later. They associate not eating breakfast with having an empty stomach, and hence with fat-burning. If they "slip" and eat, they now have license to eat whatever they want for the rest of the day and start again on "NOEP" the next day. Next comes lunch, often eaten in public. This usually consists of a salad or vegetarian platter and a diet soda or diet iced tea. Low-fat yogurt is the usual "dessert." By 5:00, all hell is breaking loose in their heads and their stomachs. Merely opening the front door at home provides the cue to raid the kitchen cabinets and refrigerator and gorge. This feeding frenzy continues after dinner, until sleep takes over. Sometimes this overeating is part of a pattern of self-reward for being so "good" and eating healthfully and in small portions all day.

Many overweight patients, even some who weigh over 400 pounds, claim that they do not eat a great deal. Researchers are skeptical, yet there are some obese patients who really do not eat a great deal. However, what I have found is that many patients don't *think* they eat a great deal because they starve themselves during the day and eat only at night. They think that if they do this, the body will burn fat during the day—they equate hunger with fat burning. The study of semi-starved soldiers cited earlier in this chapter has already taught us that in severely restricting calories, you only burn muscle and lose water. This habit of daytime deprivation would explain why, in most studies, overweight people have underestimated their calorie intake by almost 50%!

I know this pattern of overeating and denying it all too well. It's what I used to do when I weighed 250 pounds. This pattern continued until I found a better *way* to eat, without changing *what* I eat. You can do this too by . . .

Eating to Match Your Metabolism

The eating pattern described above has one consequence: It makes us heavy because it fights the body's own metabolism by setting off the alarms we discussed earlier in this chapter. Fighting your metabolism usually makes your body more adept at fat storage. Studies done with rats have indicated that eating just one meal per day can do more harm than good. In the research, rats that were fed one large meal a day gained more weight than a control group that was fed the same amount of calories, over three meals. There are studies that show that perhaps one large meal a day distends the stomach abnormally. Hormones in the stomach that tell us we are full may function incorrectly when the stomach is overburdened by one large meal. A quick review of metabolism is necessary here. Metabolism is the production of energy by all of the body's cells. In order to stay alive, we, in each of our cells, need to create energy from the food that we eat. This energy is used to power all the body's cells. It allows our eyes to see, our hearts to beat, and our bodies to move. The creation of energy in our cells gives off heat, which is measured in calories. The amount of heat (energy) we create from burning calories is our metabolic rate.

Here is a "top ten" list of facts about metabolism:

1. Metabolism varies from person to person.
2. Metabolism works 24 hours a day. We burn calories every second we are alive: at work, at play, and even while sleeping.
3. As we age, our metabolic rate slows slightly.
4. Our metabolic rate peaks around age 19.
5. Our metabolic rate is partially controlled by the thyroid gland, located in the neck.
6. The metabolic rate is higher in men than in women because of men's greater amount of muscle tissue, which burns more calories than fat.
7. Metabolism rises with fever or increased activity.
8. The metabolic rate is a function of body size. The larger your body size, the higher your metabolic rate (not the opposite, as everyone thinks!).
9. Your metabolic rate can be inherited.
10. Metabolism is biphasic, having day and night phases.

This last attribute is most important both in learning a new way to eat and in understanding the dosing of Redux. During the day, from approximately 8:00 A.M. to 7:00 P.M., our metabolisms are high. The body is in its "hot phase," awake and ready for its daily activity. You are sharp mentally, your heart is pumping strongly, and you are using your muscles to move and carry things. Now, look at what happens if you eat little or no breakfast or lunch. You artificially force the metabolic rate down because the neuropeptide Y in your hypothalamus interprets your meager caloric intake as starvation, and your body's metabolism lowers in order to conserve energy. Remember what we said about Redux not working with a very-low-calorie diet? Well, by not eating during the day, you have created a situation where Redux can't work! Your body is allowing you to eat during the day, and you're not listening! Why bother taking your morning dose of Redux if you're not going to eat anyway?

Now comes that evening feeding frenzy! It's 7:00 P.M. and your metabolic rate is slowing down as the body prepares to sleep. You aren't as sharp mentally, your heart rate is slowing, and your body is getting ready to relax. Even your digestive system has slowed down. (Interestingly, it seems only the taste buds on the tongue work best at night!) What do you do when you eat a big dinner and snack all night long? You "dump" most of your calories on a body and digestive system that are not ready to receive them. Your whole body is gearing down for its sleep mode. You know intuitively that forcing your digestive and circulatory systems to digest and metabolize food at night is not in harmony with what your body truly wants: rest! In fact, many people who eat late have problems sleeping. I have had many patients tell me that they sleep much better once they stop eating late. When you do eat late at night, the body stores many of those calories as fat.

While you sleep, instead of resting, your body works to maintain those fat stores! The word "metabolism" comes from the Greek word *metaballein*, which means "to change." This is exactly what you will have to do, by doing what I call meal reversal.

Meal Reversal

Everyone pays lip service to "changing lifestyles" and "developing healthier eating habits." If you are to be thin in this lifetime, you must act now. The easiest way to change your eating habits and get in sync with the daily rhythms of your body (called the circadian rhythms) is to make sure you eat a substantial lunch. Lunch must consist of a good protein source (fish, meat, or poultry), along with your favorite fats and carbohydrates, so that you feel satisfied after the meal and throughout the afternoon. Taking Redux in the morning (it is a medication to be taken twice a day) will help you at the beginning. You see, when you eat as I've described, you are helping Redux because you are taking in enough calories to make it work. Too much caloric restriction sets in motion the body forces that oppose weight loss. Redux cannot overcome these forces.

How much should you eat for lunch? No one knows exactly; the scale will tell you how you're doing. In any case, this is a new experience for you—so enjoy it! Redux will protect you from any large increase in fat or carbohydrate intake. Remember, all that you are asked to do each day with Redux's help is to reduce your calorie intake by 200 to 300 calories. What you are ultimately trying to accomplish is to change the biochemistry of your body. When you open that front door as you arrive home in the evening, instead of feeling starved, you will feel moderately hungry at most. Once you have mastered this pattern, begun with the help of Redux, you will be set for life. (Remember, this is something that you get better at as time goes on—it's an acquired skill. Isn't it funny how I'm begging you to eat lunch? I told you this wasn't a "diet" book!)

To complete our being in sync with our metabolisms, *a low-carbohydrate dinner, and all accompanying snacks, should be finished by 7:00—at the latest.* This matches the time when the body's metabolic rate slows. The earlier dinner ends, the better. At 7:00, all eating stops. If you usually snack on pretzels and ice cream while watching TV at 10:00, you don't have to give up your favorite snacks. The only change is *when* you can eat them, so have them for dessert! Eating by 7:00 is extremely important, as is eating a dinner low in carbohydrates. We will see exactly why this holds true in the next chapter.

A dose of Redux in the afternoon allows us not to eat a huge dinner, not to have a huge dessert, and not to snack into the night. You have now put yourself in sync with your metabolism. Doing this allows your body to metabolize the lunch you ate, and it gives your body the time it needs in the night to burn off the calories you consumed at dinner. The goal of not snacking at night is quite easy to accomplish, once you realize that you are actually consuming almost the same amount of food, almost the same number of calories, just at different times. Author and authority on weight loss Dr. Kenneth Cooper, the founder of the Cooper Aerobics Center in Dallas, has stated that he believes the obese should consume 75% of their calories before 1:00 P.M.! Don't be afraid that you may not be able to stop the late-night snacking, Redux will help you to do this.

I lost my weight by no longer "living" for dinner. It is no

longer my "refuge meal." I eat a nice lunch and am content for the rest of the day. This is what my patients do, as well. They teach themselves that it is all right to go to bed a bit hungry, if necessary. This practice of eating a good lunch and of not eating late is often followed by actors and actresses. Years ago, on *The Dinah Shore Show*, Lucille Ball confessed that she never ate dinner past 4:30 P.M.! Many of my patients love the idea and the results of the discipline they develop, and so will you! These are some of the responses I've gotten from patients:

"I don't mind not eating at night because the next day I can have what I want."

"When I eat lunch, I eat less at night."

"My husband usually comes home late. But I realize that this is about my weight loss, so when I join him for dinner, he eats and I talk."

The most interesting remark came from M.B., a single mother who works at a car dealership. She was my first patient to try the meal-reversal technique. She lost 60 pounds, and her picture is proudly displayed in my office. Some people put the first dollars they ever earned on the wall; I put M.B.'s before-and-after pictures. She said, "Not eating after 7:00 is really quite easy because it's the last eating habit we develop." This is true. While food preferences are established in early life, the habit of eating late usually begins in the teen years. It is definitely learned behavior and is not based on hunger, the way eating breakfast should be (consider that twelve or so hours or so have passed between dinner and breakfast). The abnormal eating habits of the overweight, especially the habit of not eating during the day, put stress on the body and cause it to issue strong signals of hunger. When you eat a substantial lunch and feel full afterward, you will lessen the intensity of your hunger at dinner. Of course, this process is made easier by that afternoon dose of Redux. Now you can see how you get better at this as you practice more! You actually teach your body to change biochemically!

If you go to a restaurant for dinner, try to go early. Try to eat a meal that is low in carbohydrates, and be sure to take your second dose of Redux. If you can't do any of the above, it is no big deal—just enjoy your dinner and start again the next day. Many patients have a problem in that their work schedules conflict with the no-food-after-7:00 deadline. I tell them that this deadline is so important that if they are to lose weight, they should eat at work—or even in transit if they have to! Your metabolism does not allow for much compromise on this score.

There is an interesting phenomenon that occurs with patients who work nights. One would think that they would be thin because they expend so much energy at night and raise their metabolism. Actually, they often aren't thin. The nighttime lowering of the metabolic rate occurs for them as it does for us. They sleep when their metabolic rates are high and eat when they are low. In essence, they give an indirect proof that my meal-reversal idea works: I have never seen a person who works the graveyard shift lose weight! Not one! They can't lose weight because they are going against the natural rhythm of their metabolism.

The amount of calories you save by eating to match your metabolism is not great over the short term, and keep in mind that Redux, in general, does not effect metabolism. However, over time, a transformation does take place in those who continually strive to follow this new pattern of not eating late. You teach your body discipline. *Discipline is a higher function than willpower.* Redux helps you develop this discipline because the afternoon dose will help you follow the evening directives, without feeling undue hunger. As you practice meal reversal, night by night, you will get better at it. This is the skill of weight loss. You will find that by practicing meal reversal and enhancing your metabolism (see Chapter 6), over time you will greatly diminish the amount of calories you ingest—and increase the amount of calories you burn! At first this happens because of Redux, but later it happens because of *you*. In fact, as soon as you master this technique of meal reversal, you won't even need Redux. Most of my patients have used weight-loss drugs for only a short period of time (a few months), and from then on have used them only on an as-needed basis. Minimizing the time you spend taking the drug is an important factor, considering Redux's—or any weight-loss medication's—potential for adverse side effects. As with any medication, the longer you take it, the more likely you are to experience side effects. There are also people in my practice who have successfully lost weight by meal reversal alone, without taking medication.

E.R. and R.S. are two volunteer firefighters who did not want to take medication because in their job they could be called at any time and they were afraid of making changes in their patterns of sleep (as we saw in Chapter 4, weight-loss medications can affect sleep). They consulted me before Redux was available. E.R. weighed 315 pounds and R.S., who started three months later, weighed 345 pounds. Both had voracious appetites, consuming most of their calories at dinner. By simply changing nighttime eating habits, along with the program outlined in Chapter 6, "Redux in Motion," E.R. is now down to 198 pounds and R.S. is down to 260. Both look and feel great. They will now have access to Redux to help keep the weight off, if they choose to. They are a source of pride in their community and have inspired many to follow their lead.

Below is a summary chart of what a typical day following

the routine I have outlined might look like. Weight loss would take place by a general reduction of caloric intake, based on both taking Redux and making your voluntary 200-to-300-calorie reduction at dinner, or during the day. If you follow this program, you will usually wake up hungry. This is a good sign. Until now, most of you were barely hungry in the morning because you were eating too much at night! The hunger you feel in the morning is a sign that your body needs food based on the biochemical changes that you helped to foster—congratulations! Now, breakfast should not consist of a bagel and cream cheese—this is what overweight people eat. Thin people *eat breakfast!* Breakfast can be any kind of cereal, pancakes, or french toast. Just go light on the syrup and stay away from hard cheeses. Remember as a child how much you enjoyed breakfast? Enjoy it again!

A DAY IN THE LIFE OF REDUX

WHAT YOU DO	*WHAT HAPPENS IN THE BODY*
1. Redux is taken in the early morning. The "hot" phase of metabolism begins.	**1.** The brain levels of serotonin rise and appetite is suppressed in about one hour.
2. Breakfast is eaten.	**2.** The body welcomes not being starved in the morning and rewards you with an increased sense of well-being.
3. Redux is working, suppressing the desire to snack between breakfast and lunch.	**3.** There are no added calories for the body to metabolize.
4. A substantial protein-based lunch is eaten.	**4.** Again, no starvation here. Neuropeptide Y is quiet! No increase in appetite.

5. The second dose of Redux is taken in the late afternoon.

5. Appetite suppression and decreased preoccupation with food will continue until sleep ensues.

6. Dinner is consumed before 7:00. You voluntarily cut back 200 to 300 calories of fat and carbohydrates. The "cold" phase of metabolism begins.

6. Insulin levels are kept down through the evening and night, lessening post-dinner hunger and the burden of digesting food at night. Insulin naturally falls two to three hours after eating, but you amplified this fall by not consuming a high-carbohydrate dinner. The body is now less adept at storing fat.

Well, you made it through the "food part" of *The Redux™ Revolution*. Not too bad, was it? Wait until you see what's in store for you in the next chapter.

DID YOU KNOW . . .

- 50% of all American women and 25% of all American men are on diets each day.
- Liquid diets have necessitated gallbladder surgeries and have caused deaths.
- Liquid diets still bring in $30 million per year.
- Women who retain water (that is, suffer from edema) around the time of their period can sometimes gain up to 15 pounds in water weight.
- Infants and children have higher requirements for proteins than adults and should not be on diets of any kind unless so authorized by a qualified physician.

Chapter 6

Redux in Motion

A ssisi, the birthplace of St. Francis, is one of the most beautiful spots on earth. Located in central Italy, it has remained virtually unchanged over the past 800 years. From the
promontory of Barbarosa's castle to the church of St. Francis's
confidante, St. Clare, to the basilicas of the saint himself,
which contain his relics, this city offers a spiritual experience
wherever you look. Imagine you and I are there right now,
ascending to St. Francis's favorite place of meditation—
Mount Subasio, which dominates the landscape. There we
find two brown-robed monks who inhabit a monastery. The
brothers are bound to a vow of silence. One monk sits inside
at a desk, illuminating manuscripts. The other is outside in
the sun, sweating, gathering grapes. Both are overweight. As
we sit down to lunch with them, I ask you which of the two
will be hungrier. Forget neuropeptide Y, forget leptin; give
me your honest answer, from "the gut." I have posed this

question to almost 3,000 people, and 99.9% have given the same answer you probably came up with: *The monk who is working outside is the hungriest!* The exercise he performed increased his appetite! If you are overweight, each time that *you* exercise, you do the same thing as the monk—you increase your appetite.

The expression "working up an appetite" never rang truer. At the beginning of this book, we discussed how *The Redux™ Revolution* requires a change in attitude and an open mind to new ideas. So open up to this idea: In my opinion, based on 25 years of experience and research, *exercise does not cause weight loss. In many cases, it can actually foster weight gain!*

In reality, this should not be difficult to understand, for reasons we'll discuss. Fewer than 50% of Americans exercise regularly. As for the obese, I estimate that no more than 5% to 10% exercise regularly. Many overweight people do not even try to lose weight because they fear the "exercise part" of a weight-loss plan. It is pure fantasy to suppose that millions of overweight Americans who didn't exercise when they were younger and thinner would suddenly be inspired to start jogging or bicycling when they are older and heavier. Not only is it unrealistic, but as we shall see, it could be dangerous, too! In any event, going to the gym or using a home exercise machine will not cause weight loss if you are overweight.

Before there is any misunderstanding, let me explain a few things. As a lifelong fitness enthusiast, I am not an "exercise-basher." In fact, I am an advocate of exercise—provided it is used in the proper way. In my opinion, exercise is best used for maintenance, not for initial weight loss. Exercise certainly has its place in cardiovascular fitness, muscle toning, overall good health, and feeling good about yourself. What I am saying is this: *If you are overweight, the same biochemical differences that explain why diets don't result in weight loss assume an even greater role in explaining why exercise does not cause weight loss.* I have exercised with heavy weights daily for 25 years. Not only did I never lose a single pound from weight training, but I actually gained about 40 pounds of unwanted fat. In all my years of experience, in gyms across the world, I have never seen an obese person lose weight by working out. Sure, I have seen people without a strong obesity gene lose a few pounds on a combination of diet and exercise. I have seen thin people get thinner, and some postpartum women (women who have recently given birth) shed some weight as well.

Theoretically, exercise, by burning a certain amount of calories, should cause weight loss without dieting. This can occur, only very rarely, in thin people and in top athletes. Do you know anyone who was obese who lost weight via exercise alone, with no dieting? I doubt it. Research clearly shows that exercise by itself can, at best, cause only a 5% decrease in body weight. This means that a 200-pound man can exercise and drop to 190 pounds, under ideal conditions. What about women? Women do not fare as well, because they do not have as much muscle as men. Because you need muscle to burn fat, the more muscle you have, the greater your capacity to burn fat. Women also do not have enough testosterone, the hormone needed to sustain muscle.

However, there is good news, even on this front: Redux can negate the increase in appetite that I believe exercise causes for both men and women. But first, let's examine "the body of evidence."

The Body of Evidence

There is ample scientific evidence that exercise does not cause weight loss. In general, the body looks upon exercise as the acute loss of calories. It responds by making immediate adjustments that make our appetite increase in as short a time as four to six hours. It does this in an attempt to compensate for the body's loss of calories as the result of exercise. This is what happened to the monk working outside: He worked hard, felt hungrier as a result, and ate more. So he is as overweight as the monk who sits inside all day. It happened to me, despite thousands of workouts over the years, and it probably happened to you. Here is a closer look at what actually occurs in your brain and body that counters our chances for burning calories via exercise.

There are four major weight-promoting factors that are unleashed each time you exercise: neuropeptide Y, endorphins, insulin and insulin resistance, and food preferences after exercise. We will discuss each below.

Neuropeptide Y. In Chapter 2 we learned that neuropeptide Y is a controlling protein in the brain that increases our appetite in response to dieting and exercise. The more neuropeptide Y you have, the hungrier you are and the greater your tendency to gain weight. Remember that study I cited in Chapter 2 that involved dieting and exercising mice? One conclusion that can be drawn from that study is that since neuropeptide Y levels were equally elevated when a mouse either lowers its calorie intake drastically or exercises vigorously, the mouse actually interprets exercise as starvation! The same is thought to occur in humans, who have similar changes in neuropeptide Y in response in exercise and starvation. However, it is a lot easier to study mice than people in this situation—the mice must be killed to measure the level of neuropeptide Y in their brains. Like the mice, your body is ever vigilant against a calorie restriction of any kind. Burning calories via exercise can be seen by your body as deprivation of energy. Vigorous exercise therefore becomes a key factor in elevating neuropeptide Y and appetite, eventually causing weight gain.

Endorphins. These are the neurotransmitters in the brain that have been called the "happy brain chemicals." In fact, the word "endorphin" comes from "*end*ogenous *m*orphine." Endorphins are so named because they play a role in pain perception and in the "exercise high" we feel after exercise (runners call it "runners' high"). In fact, this is why exercise is thought to be addictive. You can actually develop a need for the brain to "feel" the endorphins. The exercise high forms the basis of the exercise infomercial industry. In exercise infomercials, we see attractive, tanned, thin instructors hawking their favorite form of exercise machine. Smiling as they demonstrate how to use the machine, they talk constantly of the "great feeling" that you get from exercise. This feeling has a biochemical basis in endorphin secretion in the hypothalamus. What the instructors don't tell you is that endorphins stimulate appetite in the hypothalamus as well as in the stomach. *When you exercise, you become hungrier.* Although some studies and some patients claim that exercise curbs your appetite, this phenomenon is temporary. Your appetite may drop in the immediate post-exercise period, for 15 minutes to an hour, but then your hunger becomes unbearable. Endorphins and neuropeptide Y, your brain's two most powerful neurotransmitters, are working against you. Can it get worse? You bet. Keep reading.

Insulin and insulin resistance. In Chapter 2 we noted that the obese have high levels of insulin, which keep them hungry, and that insulin resistance prevents the insulin from working properly. When you exercise, certain hormones, like glucagon, growth hormones, and adrenaline, become elevated in the blood. Their role is to break down fat in the post-exercise period. However, insulin resistance can prevent this from happening on any large scale. In addition, the stress on the body produced by exercise can cause insulin levels, which fall during exercise, to rise even higher after exercise. This, again, makes you even hungrier than before.

Food preferences after exercise. The foods we are most likely to crave in the appetite-elevated period after exercise are fats and carbohydrates—the very foods that got us into trouble with weight in the first place!

In a study published in the *European Journal of Clinical Nutrition* in February 1995, researchers studied the food preferences of lean, healthy college students. The students were asked to run or cycle at high intensity levels. Afterward, their food intake was measured, both qualitatively and quantitatively. The researchers found that the students did not change the total amount of food they ate after exercise as compared to how much they ate when they didn't exercise, but each person craved high-fat foods, which pile on the calories! These foods totally negated any calorie expenditure resulting from the exercise itself!

Many of you would be surprised to learn that standard textbooks on internal medicine and the medical literature on obesity also have divergent views on exercise as a mode of weight loss. I know I was! The texts imply that exercise is not a good way to lose weight, and that it can cause an increase in appetite. In the Bibliography, I cite references for those of you who would like to research this further. Multiple studies with rats have shown that increasing activity can increase appetite in female rats. Studies also have shown that exercise has different effects on those who are sedentary and on those who are not. Research on sedentary individuals shows that exercise can decrease appetite, whereas in active individuals, exercise has proved to increase appetite! Incidentally, if you work outside the home, go to school, or take care of children, you are not considered sedentary. Sedentary, in these studies, means a 12-hour "couch potato." Fortunately, few of us would qualify.

The sum total of these findings, in my opinion, is that the effect of exercise on weight loss is not a beneficial one. There are only two kinds of people who exercise: those who are in shape and those who will never be! Now comes the real zinger. You might be thinking, "If I want to be healthy, doesn't exercise help my heart?" The answer to this question comes from a remarkable study that was featured in the December 27, 1995, issue of the *Journal of the American Medical Association*. The study included research done at the Maryland School of Medicine, the VA Hospital in Baltimore, and the National Institutes of Health. These studies took 170 obese middle-aged and older men and separated them into three groups. One group did aerobic exercise for 45-minute intervals three times a week and were fed so that no weight loss would occur for nine months. A second group went on a calorie-restricted diet for nine months and lost weight. The third group, the control group, was instructed not to lose weight or change their diets. After this time, all groups' cardiac risk factors—including blood pressure, insulin levels, cholesterol levels, high-density-lipoprotein (HDL) levels, and glucose levels—were tested. To the surprise of researchers, all of the cardiac risk factors had changed favorably in the weight-loss group, while only a few changes, all with lesser magnitude, occurred in the exercise group! The average weight loss in the 44 men in the weight-loss group who completed the study was 20 pounds. This proves the premise that even slight weight loss can bring about improvement in health. This study received national attention, including a large article in the *New York Times* with the headline "Study Says Weight Loss Beats Exercise to Lower Health Risks." It turns out that exercise isn't even that beneficial for the one thing for which it is touted so highly: to improve our cardiovascular fitness level! Weight loss increased cardiovascular health when exercise did not!

But aren't exercise and fitness synonymous with health? No. For those of you who watched the Superbowl this past January, did you notice the size of those linemen? It seemed that every five minutes or so, the announcers were telestrating some lineman's prodigious belly—extolling their girth! These men are physically fit. They get paid millions of dollars to move their bulk around rather rapidly. Each can do the 40-yard run in a few seconds. Yet all of these men face the same health risks as anyone who is obese. In fact, as we said in Chapter 1, since these men are mostly apple-shaped, they are prime candidates for diabetes, high blood pressure, and other obesity-related disorders. These men are *not* healthy.

If only five out of every 100 obese persons exercise, why bother with this discussion in the first place? Why am I trying to convince people who don't exercise that exercise is not that important? Ah, but it is! Remember, I stated I am an advocate for exercise when it is used in the right way. If you want to keep weight off forever, exercise is a great tool for maintenance! Once you lose the weight with Redux's help and get healthy, use exercise to keep the weight off and stay healthy!

Metabolic Makeover: The Final Body Rule

In Chapter 5, we learned how to lose weight in a way that would keep the metabolism as high as possible, with as little muscle loss as possible. Now I will show you how Redux and an entirely new concept in raising your metabolism can help you to lose weight permanently. Traditional exercise does not cause weight loss, but exercise can help lose weight and keep it off, once you learn the final Body Rule.

Redux has the power to change all the negative things I've just said about exercise. If you take Redux and decide to exercise, the medication can, in my opinion, block the increased appetite caused by elevated neuropeptide Y, endorphins, and insulin resistance, which, we have noted, rise in response to the body's perception that it is being starved of calories when you exercise. With Redux, you will burn calories with only positive results.

I discourage my patients from exercising while they are trying to lose weight, unless they are on medication. The medicine serves as a wonderful "equalizer" and allows their bodies to function just like those of thin people. Obese people can now exercise and lose weight. Here, Redux works to correct a most unfair biochemical disadvantage!

I should know. I had exactly that disadvantage. For the past eight years, I have been trying to elevate only one person's metabolism—mine! As I said previously, I had gained much fat despite constant exercise. I had competed as a bodybuilder and as a power lifter, even placing third in my class in the 1992 Drug Free World II Bench Press Championships. Yet, I wanted to be thinner. Four years ago, because of new work demands, I had to stop weight-lifting for a two-month period.

113

Fortunately, during this time, I came home earlier and ate before 6:30. I decided to do push-ups and sit-ups before bed, in an effort to keep up my muscle tone. To my surprise, I lost ten pounds over those two months. When I went back to weight-lifting, I gained all the weight back in just four weeks. It didn't make sense—or did it? What had I been overlooking? Utilizing hospital computers, I did extensive research on exercise and weight loss, and on metabolism and exercise. What I learned astounded me! All along, my weight-lifting had been fueling an ever-increasing desire to eat! With a father and a grandmother who were diabetics, I was a classic "Syndrome X-er." I was fat and getting fatter. But no more. I now weigh 190 pounds at 6'2". I can bench-press twice my body weight and can squat three times my weight. These figures match those of most NFL linebackers—and I am 46 years old. The secret to my success is what I call "natural liposuction."

Natural Liposuction

Suppose I told you that there is a perfect exercise, and a perfect time to do this exercise, that will raise your metabolic rate and help keep weight off. This one exercise will accomplish all that running many miles does—but without all the pain and sweat! You can even do this exercise without leaving your chair.

In the previous chapter, we learned that it is best to be finished with dinner no later than 7:00 P.M., out of respect for our falling metabolism. Let's take a look at what happens in our bodies in the evening. Insulin levels, already high in the obese, rise even higher after dinner. This is to help metabolize the carbohydrates we ate at dinner. To lower the magnitude of this insulin response, we have already decided on a low-carbohydrate dinner, if possible. Time passes: 7:00, 8:00, 8:30. Insulin levels are going down and will remain as low as possible through the night, as long as we don't snack. Now is the perfect time to exercise, because the hormones that burn fat—glucagon, growth hormone, adrenaline, and cortisol—only come out to play when insulin levels go down! Your body is now ready to burn fat; are *you*? Any exercise you do now, at least 2½ hours after your last meal, will essentially burn fat and raise your metabolism. This happens because when you exercise, you utilize glycogen, the sugar stored in the muscles.

If you don't eat between dinner and exercise, and you don't eat after exercise, you allow your body to do what it is supposed to do: It can now take fat from wherever you have it, bring it to a muscle, and have the enzymes in your muscle turn that fat to sugar. Your body chips away at fat deposits on the abdomen, thighs, and hips. It sends those deposits up to any muscle that you used during exercise. This conversion is a form of "natural liposuction." This process takes hours to complete and requires energy, which raises your metabolism. Moreover, you are raising your metabolism at a time when it's usually at its lowest—when you sleep. You don't feel anything. The body automatically burns fat, even when we sleep. Each night that you eat and exercise as I will describe, you burn more fat. By the way, you can have as much water, diet soda, or any drink that does not contain calories as you wish, when you finish exercising. Any calories you ingest at this point would replace the sugar you utilized when you exercised, without ever getting to your fat reserves.

Exercise, done at any other time of day, does not burn large amounts of fat. If you want to exercise in the morning, as I used to, you burn mostly glycogen (unless you are a top athlete). This glycogen is the body's storage form of sugar and would be quickly replaced by any carbohydrates you consumed at breakfast. Thus, your morning exercise results in minimal calorie (and weight) loss. The best time to accomplish this metabolic boost is at night. At night, you can't stimulate your appetite for food because you'll be sleeping! Remember, it's not only *how* you exercise, it's *when* you exercise!

Now that you know the best time to exercise, what are the best exercises? The following is a list of ten popular exercises, from the most efficient—those that burn the most calories and use the most energy in the least time—to the least efficient. The list may surprise you.

1. Circuit weight training
2. Aerobic dancing
3. Cross-country skiing
4. Jogging
5. Swimming
6. Cycling
7. Tennis
8. Gardening
9. Golfing
10. Walking

We all think of walking as the ideal exercise—but it isn't. In fact, walking is the least efficient total-body exercise you can do if you want to lose weight. *If people continue to walk for exercise, they will remain overweight.* Not only does walking burn a relatively small amount of calories, but it also stimulates appetite! This is a poor prescription for weight loss. Surprisingly, walking burns the fewest amount of calories of any human activity that involves total-body motion! Gardening burns more calories than walking at a moderate pace. It's amazing that doctors still advise patients to walk in order to lose weight.

The real problem we have is not walking, but rather timing. If the best time to exercise is at least 2½ hours after you last eat, won't you be too tired to do any form of exercise—especially on an empty stomach? Looking at our list, we see that the top two exercises are circuit weight training and aerobic dancing. Circuit training is defined as the constant movement of a muscle group against resistance—i.e., weight-lifting. Both of these exercises burn about 2.5 times the calories that moderately intense walking does. Circuit training and aerobic dancing are the perfect exercises for both the evening couch potato and those who are more ambulatory. Let's look at aerobic dancing first. If a person does 15 minutes of aerobic dancing, 2½ hours after eating, this is the equivalent of walking for 35 minutes. (Keep in mind that it is crucial that no food be eaten after exercise.) The combination of aerobic dancing without food in the stomach activates the body's metabolism-elevating mechanism. Aerobic dancing in this way must be done at least four nights a week, and if you increase the frequency, or exercise more vigorously or for longer durations, you increase the calorie-burning process. If you don't feel like doing aerobic dancing, you can dance fast in a sustained fashion to your favorite music for half an hour.

As long as you wait to exercise at least 2½ hours after your last meal, any exercise you do will burn calories and raise your metabolic rate until morning. You can now use that exercise machine you ordered; you can wipe the dust off your NordicTrack and put it to work. The only difference is that these methods will now work for you by burning calories through the night—without increasing appetite.

Circuit weight training is still the best method for burning calories in the way I've described. Since many of us sit and watch TV at night, why not use this time wisely? All you need to do is pick up a dumbbell (three to five pounds for women and five to ten pounds for men) and move it continuously for at least 15 minutes in the form of shoulder presses, lateral raises, bicep curls, and wrist curls.

If you have done weight training, you know what these exercises are. Those of you who may not have done weight training can either go to the library and check out a book on weight training, or ask a qualified trainer at your local gym. The key in successful circuit weight training is to keep the weight moving at all times, alternating exercises and body parts. Do not count repetitions. You should be paying attention to the TV, because dumbbell movements are to be done while sitting and watching TV! Remember what we said about "natural liposuction." We aren't trying to build muscles; we are trying to make them more efficient fat burners! In doing these weight-training movements, or in doing aerobic exercise, you literally "suck" the fat out of cells. You then transform that fat into sugar in the very muscles you just used to exercise. The more you do it, the better your body gets at it. A study published in the 1993 *Journal of Applied Physiology* found that the metabolic rate in people who exercise as with dumbbells as I've described was 9% higher than in those who didn't—even 15 hours after the weight workout! The group in the study actually burned more calories after exercise than during it. Your muscles will become potent fat burners. Your metabolic makeover will be complete!

I would like to briefly address a concern that many women have about weight training: fear of becoming muscle-bound. Nothing could be further from the truth! Believe it or not, the heavier you are, the more muscle you already have! Nature provides the extra muscle to move around a larger bulk.

In general, women do not build big muscles because you need testosterone to do so and women have only trace amounts of testosterone in their bodies. In any case, the dumbbell movements prescribed above do not cause muscles to get larger. Rather, they coax the muscle to do what we want it to: suck out some body fat and use it as fuel! They will also shape the muscles for a trimmer look.

Redux: The Magic Pill for Exercise

Redux plays two key roles in making exercise finally work for you. First, it blocks the appetite-increasing effects of exercise, should you decide to exercise during the day. You can now use exercise as a true weight-loss tool. Second, it will help you to establish the habit of not eating in the evening. It is extremely important that you not eat after exercising. On occasion, it's permissible to have a small snack, between 100 and 150 calories, in between dinner and exercise. It is best, though, to avoid this practice. The only way many of you can abstain from your evening eating practice is by taking that afternoon dose of Redux and turning those thoughts of food to thoughts of exercise. Of course, this plan still works without Redux. If you decide not to take Redux, follow the rest of the program, as I have outlined it, and you will lose weight. The only exercise you must do is 15 minutes of weight training at least 2½ hours after dinner. You do not have to increase your heart rate, you do not have to sweat. Just make sure you put at least moderate effort into it. *Be sure to consult your doctor before beginning exercise of any kind. Many cardiac patients can do weight training under medical supervision.*

When you combine the eating program from Chapter 5 with the exercise program outlined in this chapter, there is a synergistic effect on the metabolism. It stays as high as nature will allow. I firmly believe that the only way to keep weight off is to keep your metabolism as high as possible from day one of your weight-loss efforts. Redux helps make this happen.

With or without Redux, there is no point to taking weight off if you are not prepared to defend your new weight with a little effort. Now that you are terrific at taking weight off, how do you think you'll be at keeping it off? Is there life after Redux? Read on.

DID YOU KNOW . . .

- The more you weigh, the more calories you burn doing the same exercise as a thinner person.
- 98% of all fat that is burned is burned in muscle.
- Studies have shown that octogenarians can get stronger with weight training.
- People who engage in weight-lifting develop thicker bones and are less likely to get osteoporosis—a bone-thinning disease seen most often in postmenopausal women.
- There are women power lifters who can bench-press close to 400 pounds.
- Intense exercise can affect the menses adversely.
- Muscles burn fat when they rest and sugar when they exercise.
- According to Dr. Frank Lattarulo, a podiatrist in Westchester, New York, when an obese person runs, the ground can exert a force of seven times the body weight on the foot—for a 250-pound person, this is a force of 1,750 pounds!

Chapter 7

Life After Redux

It has been about eight weeks since you started taking Redux. Weight loss is progressing smoothly. You are becoming accustomed to the new meal reversal pattern described in Chapter 5, and the evening exercises have become habit. You are noticeably less hungry; the usual cues that used to prompt dashes to the refrigerator no longer have power over you. Your internal food dialogue is distant, barely intelligible.

As you reflect on your success, you feel pangs of self-doubt, recollecting past dietary failures. After all, you may have reached this level of weight loss before, even exceeded it, perhaps more than once. Yet you always regained any lost weight. Why should this weight-loss episode be any different?

If Redux has an answer to the national weight-loss dilemma, that answer must come in the form of a viable maintenance program. We begin with this premise: *There is no reason even to attempt weight loss with Redux unless you have a plan to keep the weight off.* This book provides such a plan.

Many researchers have likened obesity to hypertension. Both are chronic medical problems that require daily medication on an indefinite basis. Research scientists and clinicians therefore advocate taking either Redux or phen/fen on an ongoing basis, even after weight loss has ceased. Thus, Redux would serve as a medication of maintenance. Two problems arise with this approach. First, there are no studies to confirm the safety of taking Redux for longer than one year. While it is true that Redux has been used in Europe for ten years, there are unfortunately no studies to prove either safety or efficacy for that long a period of time. Until there are safety confirmations for use longer than one year, and until the issue of PPH (primary pulmonary hypertension; see Chapter 4) is resolved, it is my opinion that it is still premature to assume that Redux should be used on a daily basis for more than a few months at a time. Secondly, there are no studies to show that Redux works in large patient populations beyond one year.

Does this mean that Redux and other weight-loss medications are not going to help us keep weight off at all? After all, this is the very reason we need medication in the first place! Yes, Redux and phen/fen will help with permanent weight loss, because *The Redux™ Revolution* offers a fresh, dynamic approach to weight-loss maintenance that flexes and bends to meet your lifestyle.

Time Capsule

It has always surprised me how many patients who have lost weight have gone on to do nothing to keep the weight off.

They do not defend their new weight. Suppose you suddenly came into possession of the most exotic and expensive sports car. Wouldn't you pamper it? Wouldn't you shine it, wax it, and protect it? Yet many people who lose weight do not apply this same level of care to their bodies, even though they worked hard to attain their new figures. It's as if they believe that the weight should stay off by itself, just because they have worked so hard to lose it. Unfortunately, nothing could be further from the truth.

The key to keeping weight off lies in understanding what is known as the body's set point. The set point is a weight that your body seems to rally around. Your body does everything it can to maintain this body weight by lowering metabolism and increasing appetite. If you have lost weight in the past, you probably know what your set point is, within two or three pounds. It is the "sticking point" in weight loss that is more powerful than a mere plateau. You just can't seem to lose weight after reaching it. In fact, your weight-loss victories only give the body more impetus to maintain the set point you had *before* you lost weight.

The set point, or "adipostat," is a fat-sensing thermostat that is located mostly, but not completely, in the hypothalamus. Its chief role is in maintaining our fat stores. Leptin is the hormone that lets the brain know how much fat is stored in the body. It exerts its action on various sites in the hypothalamus, influencing the set point and production of neuropeptide Y. It is presumed that in nonoverweight individuals, leptin levels fall in proportion to the amount of fat lost. In the obese, the amount of leptin falls at a greater rate than the rate of fat lost. Remember, as leptin levels fall, the levels of neuropeptide Y in the hypothalamus increase. Neuropeptide Y, insulin, and various other hormones are the chief effectors of increased appetite. The obese, therefore, are even more disadvantaged with weight loss when compared to their thinner counterparts, because their greater rate of leptin loss triggers a more extreme increase in neuropeptide Y, which triggers hunger. The set point "senses," presumably from loss of leptin, that fat stores are being depleted. When this occurs, the hypothalamus sends out a signal, the exact nature of which is unknown. This signal tells the brain that the metabolism should be slowed and appetite increased. When this occurs, your weight-loss efforts are essentially finished. At this point, your whole body goes full steam into a weight-gain mode.

Unlike neuropeptide Y, the set point does not act right away. It is far more insidious. It can take weeks, months, or even years to jump to action. Worse yet, your set point, in general, sets itself at a higher level as you age, disposing you to gain weight later in life. In fact, the "yo-yo" effect is actually the set point setting itself higher each time you lose weight. This means that your next weight-loss attempt would be thwarted even sooner than before! There are, however, three ways to lower the set point:

- Weight-loss medication
- Cutting back on calories from fat
- Habitual exercise

Lowering the adipostat by implementing the three factors above is the backbone of *The Redux™ Revolution*'s maintenance program. We want to use these three elements to exert constant positive pressure on the set point. Under positive pressure, the set point will reset itself at a lower level that allows for easier and greater weight loss over time. It also makes it more difficult to regain any of the weight lost! Maintenance with *The Redux™ Revolution* begins with modifying the relationship between time and weight loss. My patients know that I cringe when successful before-and-after pictures are shown, and the first question asked is "How long did it take?" My response is always the same: "Who cares?" The most important question should be "How long has this person kept the weight off?" You should know by now that the body has a predetermined rate of weight loss. While this rate varies among different people, any weight lost faster than this individualized rate means that too much muscle is being lost, and muscle loss sets you up for inevitable failure—a victory for your body and its set point. In Chapter 5, we spent some time reviewing the importance of slowing the initial rate of weight loss. Now you know why: We want to keep neuropeptide Y and the set point quiet! They maintain a perennial 24-hour watch over our fat stores, as well as our muscle mass. Losing muscle mass is interpreted by neuropeptide Y and the set point as "highway robbery," almost to the same extent as losing too much fat. By now, you know what this leads to: the great weight-loss dead end!

People trying to lose weight seem to believe that the only way to achieve weight loss is by trying to race against some internal clock. It seems as if they are on a quest to lose as many pounds as possible by a certain date, because weight loss slows eventually, and they want to lose as much weight as possible before that happens. But as we have seen, rapid weight loss only triggers the slowdown (and the regain) sooner.

The Redux Revolution gives you another option. Today, right now, should be the best time in your life to lose weight. You are younger than you are ever going to be; hence your body has less of a tendency to deposit fat today than it will tomorrow. This means that in all probability, you weigh less today than you will one year from now. Your body's rate of fat deposition as you grow older is a function of the obesity gene, neuropeptide Y, high insulin levels, and changes in metabolism. However, it is also a function of your eating habits and activity levels. The Redux Revolution proposes that you alter your internal biochemical makeup to put yourself in a weight-loss mode—now and for the rest of your life. This means that each day you must do something either to slow the deposition of fat or to increase the amount of fat you "burn." The clichés of "taking each day as it comes" or "living from day to day" ring very true for people trying to lose weight. You must be prepared at all times to defend your new body weight.

When you commit yourself to defending your new body weight, Redux can exert its real power: that of "buying you time" to teach yourself the proper amount of food intake and nocturnal exercise you need to keep weight off. Suppose you weigh 220 pounds and have the desire to weigh 140 pounds. If a pill were created that could remove all that weight in 24 hours, you would be the happiest person alive—for 24 hours. You see, your body's internal biochemical structure would still be that of a 220-pound person. Your set point would be unchanged and your insulin levels still high. As the days passed, the body would realize that you had rapidly lost muscle mass and your fat stores were now depleted. This is starvation! The leptin signal would now be grossly diminished, because the fat in the fat cells producing it would have been lost. This would result in escalating levels of neuropeptide Y. Because of these events, and a stingy set point, your metabolism would be slowed while your appetite would be increased! All the while, high insulin levels would assure that you still have the hunger of a 220-pound person. Over time, you must obey these weight-gaining forces, and you would once again find yourself at 220 pounds—if you were lucky.

The set point, as we said before, often sets itself at a higher weight after a drastic weight loss. You might actually find yourself weighing 230 to 240 pounds! In essence, all that "magic pill" would have done would be to make you a 140-pound person trapped in a 220-pound eating machine of a body.

To show you how powerful your internal weight retention factors are, consider this. You are asked in this book to "voluntarily" cut back 200–300 calories per day. This does not seem like a large number of calories. If you could actually voluntarily stop eating 200–300 calories per day, all your weight-loss problems would be solved. Even if you do this only three times a week, you would still lose substantial amounts of weight over time. But until now, you couldn't do this, because your body doesn't want you to! With Redux, it will, or at least it won't mind as much. By suppressing your appetite and allowing you to initially lose weight without drastic calorie restriction, Redux enables you to begin eating as a lighter person and to do without difficulty the evening exercise I've recommended.

Set-Point Eating

Portion control of high-fat foods is another key to lowering the set point. The only way to attain portion control is for you to set your own limits, not to have someone else set them for you. Having someone else set your limits causes resentment. You are looking to use discipline, one of the higher cerebral functions we discussed in Chapter 3. Imagine your favorite Hollywood star is coming to your house for dinner. In your zeal, you prepare mountains of high-calorie food. Would you be at all surprised to find that your guest didn't eat the whole mountain, and that a certain amount of the food kept him or her satisfied? I doubt you would. Yet, you expect yourself to eat all that is put in front of you.

Research has shown that overweight people tend to consume whatever amount is put on their plates. If you are served 25 french fries, you eat 25; if you are served 15, you eat 15! Redux will allow you to feel full on 15, but *you must begin by making a conscious disciplined choice to have only 15*. Disciplined decision builds on disciplined decision. As you lose weight, slowly, your insulin levels start to come down and you feel less hungry than before. Of course, you can't defeat your own body every meal of every day. Sometimes we "let" our bodies win with overconsumption of food, but most times you win. As time goes on, you develop confidence in your own diet and in your ability to control your appetite. *For you to be successful at long-term weight loss, you must learn some degree of portion control.* This is based on the very simple idea that, activity levels aside, people who weigh less eat less than heavier people.

Research has shown that fatty foods are most appealing because of their taste. As humans, we enjoy the taste and feel in our mouth of fat. Unfortunately, past research has also shown that it is high-fat foods that lead to increased weight. Lately, however, a new and disturbing element in the American diet seems to have replaced high-fat foods as the chief culprit in weight gain: the high-carbohydrate, low-fat snack! Virtually all of my patients eat too many pretzels and low-fat bread, cakes, and cookies as snacks. It seemed like a good idea at the beginning: exchange fat, which has nine calories per gram, for carbohydrates, which have four calories per gram. However, keep in mind that at any given body weight and activity level, the amount of calories taken in each day is more or less a constant. Suppose a 200-pound woman needs 2,100 calories to "get by" each day. She goes on a stringent low-fat diet. The body, in its wisdom, knows that it still needs 2,100 calories. These calories will come from the foods our dieter is now eating: low-fat bread, low-fat pretzels, and other "healthy" snacks. As far as weight loss is concerned, it's a wash: For all the calories she is consuming in low-fat snacks, she might as well just eat a big bowl of ice cream each night—a beloved treat that she gave up when she embarked on her diet. The net result is that not only didn't our dieter lose any weight, but she is now craving the ice cream!

On the other hand, many of our favorite fatty foods are attached to carbohydrates, as is the case with cookies, cakes, and ice cream. Therefore, we must be vigilant each time we eat meals that contain fats and carbohydrates. When you sit down to a meal, try to envision what portion size a person of your *goal weight* eats. You see, every person eats some sort of "junk" food each day, only the proportions vary. Do not for one moment think that people who weigh 120 pounds don't eat cake, cookies, and ice cream. They do. They just eat less of them.

You, too, must learn portion control with the help of Redux. You will stop feeling constantly preoccupied with food, and when you do think of food, you will not only think about what types of food you like, but also about how much you will eat.

The Redux™ *Revolution*'s concept of portion control is important to master. It takes practice and it takes time. With the help of Redux, you can . . .

Become a Weight-Loss Virtuoso

In Chapter 1, we said that weight loss is a skill, like playing the piano. What is it that makes one person better at a skill than another person? First, consider underlying talent level. This may be hereditary, just as musical talent can be hereditary. In weight-loss terms, the degree of inborn ability to lose weight can be thought of as the dividing line between Pencils and Zeppelins.

Zeppelins, as we discussed in Chapter 2, have more fat cells and a greater expression of the obesity gene than Pencils. They also have higher insulin levels to keep them hungry. Therefore, they usually have less "natural" weight-loss talent than a Pencil, who has fewer fat cells, less expression of the obesity gene, and lower insulin levels and would naturally have an easier time losing weight. Portion control for Zeppelins should be extremely modest at first, relying more on Redux than on their own ability to forgo larger portions.

After natural talent comes the expertise that is born of practice. The greatest talent can only go so far without lifelong practice. The analogy here for weight loss is crystal clear: Portion control must be practiced daily. Not with *every* food choice—you "pick your spots." A bit less ice cream here, somewhat fewer cookies there. Remember, you are being helped by Redux, so the choices are quite easy to make— just make sure they are conscious decisions. Over time, as you hone your weight-loss talent, an amazing thing happens. *You acquire a new skill: a weight-loss skill.*

The exact opposite effect occurs when you buy a prepackaged meal or follow any diet plan that is not your own. You do not attain any skill level by doing these things—it's like playing a player piano! It's the conscious, repetitive eating choices that you make in a specific situation that give rise to skill. For instance, many patients find that after they try not eating at night for several consecutive nights, they no longer crave their evening snacks. This happens when they're taking weight-loss medication, and when it is stopped as well. Try doing the dumbbell movements instead of snacking for a few nights and you'll see!

While you are acquiring your skill in reducing your portions, Redux is bearing the brunt of your weight-loss burden. But soon this will change. Redux can and should be stopped. When should it be stopped? To answer this important question, let's take a step back and look at what we are trying to accomplish. Virtuoso pianists play the piano seemingly without effort because, over time, by constant practice, they fortify the neural connections between the upper part of the brain and the muscles that enable them to move the keys. The connection between the brain and the fingers takes place via neurotransmitters and relay nerves. With more practice, the part of the upper brain that controls the fine movements of the fingers becomes more adept at sending signals to the pianist's hands. The fingers themselves send back signals to the brain, via neurotransmitters, that the piano playing is proceeding well, and to continue sending the original signal to play. The more the pianist plays, the better he or she gets at playing. The same scenario can exist for people who are trying to lose weight! By using disciplined portion control, you are constantly reinforcing the cerebral cortex's ultimate control over the eating center of the hypothalamus. The hypothalamus will receive fewer pro-eating signals from the cortex, and you are on your way to accomplishing permanent weight loss! This process might take longer for a Zeppelin than for a Pencil, but both groups have similar potential mechanisms for ultimate appetite control. This change in cerebral circuitry probably is not a direct effect of Redux—which is good, because we want this process to persist after the medication is stopped. Redux gives you the biochemical opportunity to *develop your own* weight-maintenance mechanism.

A study done in Holland and published in the February

1994 edition of the *Nutrition Reviews* demonstrates how Redux should be used to help you make the transition to your new eating behavior. This study examined Redux's ability to cause weight loss over time, in a group of patients taking Redux who also adopted healthier eating styles by using portion control for fats and carbohydrates. The researchers found that over a 14-month period, the group that did not take Redux was unable to maintain their new portion-control eating habits, and they regained any weight that was lost. The group that took Redux during the first six months were able to maintain a weight loss based on portion control, even at 14 months. Researchers felt that Redux made it easier initially to stay with the program, so that the thoughts about food and feelings of deprivation commonly associated with weight loss would not sabotage weight loss over time—even when Redux was stopped.

Phase the Music

I utilize a three-phase program when using weight-loss medications.

Phase I. During this phase, twice-daily use of the medication is required. This sets the tone for initial weight-loss success, without stress. Here you begin to teach yourself portion control and you begin the meal-reversal and the evening metabolism-raising mechanisms outlined in Chapter 5. Once you start getting the hang of it and slightly modifying old habits, as outlined, you have begun the cerebral reinforcement process we have just discussed. This happens unconsciously and is a "perk" that our body gives us for practicing discipline. This phase can take from a week to two months.

In my practice, Phase I patients see me for a follow-up visit every two weeks. Once a patient tells me that he or she is following the plan and starting to lose urges to overeat, we begin Phase II (see below). I do not use the attainment of a specific weight goal as an indicator for switching phases, for a very simple reason: The important behavioral changes we have discussed have nothing at all to do with the amount of weight lost. It is not as if you will lose weight faster by being more zealous about following the plan. In fact, given what you now know about the set point, you probably realize that overdoing the plan may cause weight gain. Your reward, once you learn how to exercise portion control and follow the evening directives discussed in Chapter 5, will be to start taking less medicine.

Incidentally, many patients tell me that the medication works so well that they don't even feel like eating. They ask me if they should "force" a lunch or a dinner. I tell them no, they should never force any food intake. However, if they allow the drug to overwhelm their ability to learn portion control, they will not be able to sustain their weight loss later on, when they have stopped taking the medication. With this caveat in mind, all patients are encouraged to eat, though not to force themselves to do so.

Phase II. In this phase, we start experimenting by cutting out the morning dose. Obviously, you lessen the risks of side effects by halving the day's total dosage, but that's only part of the reason why we stop the morning dose. Remember, we are trying to encourage people to "push" more of their caloric intake to the front part of the day—breakfast and lunch. For many of you, breakfast is either eaten or not eaten out of habit. Breakfast is not a major player for us, but lunch is! *The Redux™ Revolution* encourages a large protein-anchored meal, so as to take the pressure off the body to eat a large dinner. This reversal of the usual eating pattern of the overweight is vital for long-term success!

Since we are trying to promote eating at a time when people usually don't eat, I find it best to advise patients to "ease" into lunch, adding new and more food each week at lunchtime until they feel less hungry at dinner. At this point we do not want or need Redux to suppress our appetite for lunch; we want to cultivate our appetite for lunch!

In Phase II, patients really begin to understand how their bodies are complying with their evening food intake deadline of 7:00 P.M. and their routine of evening exercises. They start actually to enjoy the discipline. At this point, many patients claim to have feelings of euphoria because they feel they are taking control of their appetite. Many patients are unsure whether it's they or the medication that is fostering this feeling of self-satisfaction. I stress that it is most definitely they! Remember: *No weight-loss medication is superior to the person taking it!* Patients can also experiment with skipping the evening dose, on occasion. It's amazing how many people can actually stop snacking at night once they have given their body an eating deadline and have followed it for a period of time! At this point, patients often tell me that they have stopped the drug of their own accord. While some patients claim they still need the medication, many more say they don't. Remember, these phases have nothing to do with time elapsed or pounds lost. Some patients can move on to Phase III very quickly, even within three or four weeks of beginning Phase II. Others may take several months. Like the rate of weight loss itself, this pace varies with each individual.

Phase III. This is essentially the phase you will be in for the rest of your life. I call it the surveillance phase. Each of us has certain cues that facilitate our overeating, or bingeing. Each patient has his or her own cues. These cues are linked to certain foods. For instance, many males in our society think of drinking beer when watching a sporting event on television. Advertisers are aware of this linkage, and that is why an inordinate amount of beer advertisements appear during the Super Bowl, stock car races, boxing matches, and the like. The cue, then, is a televised sporting event, and the associated food is beer. For many women, being able to relax after a long day of tending to work and family by watching a favorite TV show is the cue that triggers craving for a high-carbohydrate snack, like ice cream or doughnuts.

Contrary to what you may believe, these types of situations are easy to control. First, identify your cue. It's probably the one that "gets" you every night! Next, recognize that you are making a link between an external cue and food. This may have been an unconscious association that you are now bringing to conscious awareness. Now begin training yourself to work against the cue by eating that snack within the evening time frame permitted—before 7:00. You are asserting positive control.

There is, however, one cue that is hard to identify and hard to treat: boredom! The number of patients who tell me that the urge to eat when they are bored is overwhelming. However, I think that boredom must be looked at in context. Why is it that, in general, thin people do not seem to eat when they are bored, as overweight people seem to do? It is strange that the overweight never seem to knit blankets, read books, or go for walks when they are bored; it seems the cue of boredom is always linked to food intake of some sort. In my opinion, it's either their high levels of insulin that drive overweight people to eat and they target boredom as the reason, or perhaps they are depressed and are masking it with feelings of boredom. Depression will be addressed in more detail in Chapter 9. The answer I give all my patients when they tell me that they eat out of boredom is this: Look at yourself in the mirror. Are you bored, or are you depressed? If you are depressed, then that issue should be addressed by the appropriate health professional. If you are bored, combat it with a hobby that doesn't involve any sort of food intake.

With all these external cues out there, you have to keep an eye on your body every single day. You must be as vigilant against the set point as it is against you. In Phase III, the drug should be used very little, varying from once every two or three days, in the evening, to none at all. By this time, you have grasped the idea of losing weight the "correct" way and it's working for you. You are no longer in a race with yourself to lose weight, or racing with others around you.

Phen/fen, the drug regimen of choice before Redux's release, is indicated for only three months. Accordingly, in general, Phase III should begin 90 days after beginning the program. In reality, though, it's still a functional decision: What is the patient's ability to control his or her appetite after 90 days? Some patients are able to achieve appetite control in that time, while others need more time and more help. An individual's initial weight and whether a person is a Pencil or a Zeppelin are also factors. Heavier people need more time, but even for them, success depends on how well they do in following the program as outlined.

Redux has been approved for use over one year; however, I plan to reevaluate each patient after three months, not so much to check on weight loss, but to determine his or her level of appetite control. I ask my patients keep a small drug diary, and this helps to give me some idea of how they are doing. In the diary, patients log how often they are using the drug, what time of day they use it, and when and if they are hungry at all. The drug diary alerts me to some common problems that need to be addressed. For instance, many patients describe losing control over their eating when they go to barbecues in the summer or to dinner parties in the winter. I tell them to take a dose of the medication an hour or two before going out. This will give them the special protection they need when discipline is challenged. Another common problem is travel. "What should I eat when I go to Florida?" I tell all my patients to enjoy themselves and even if they have been off the medication for a while, to take it with them and use it as described above. I suggest this because the unfamiliar circumstances of a vacation can overcome any newly acquired food discipline.

By Phase III, my patients essentially have become their own weight-loss doctors. At this point, in my practice, I ask them to follow up with me as they feel they need to. Zeppelins usually take more than three months before they can be "released to their own weight-loss ability," but they are usually self-sufficient in six to eight months. It's all a matter of training!

Having been off the drug intermittently in Phase II, patients in Phase III already know how it feels to be drug-free and know that they can handle it. Once they stop the medication, I recommend that they take the drug on an as-needed basis only, like during the Christmas holiday season. Remember, when you are in Phase III you not only know about appetite control, you also know what external cues make you eat. Holidays are times when you'll be in situations that are not conducive to the surveillance of your new weight. Take the drug for a few days, or just prior to a party. During times of "body stress," such as when there are problems at work or at home, use the drug for a few days to get you over the temptation of eating in response to stress.

137

Women can experience weight gain just prior to their periods. This is part of the premenstrual syndrome, or PMS. The weight gain can occur for two reasons. First, fluid in the body can build up because of premenstrual changes in the capillary walls. Under the influence of female hormones, water leaks out of these tiny blood vessels in the hands and feet. As a result, edema, or excess water, can form in these areas. This is often noticed when shoes or rings that ordinarily fit become too tight.

Premenstrual weight gain occurs for a second reason. The appetite is actually stimulated by the hormonal changes of PMS. There is some scientific evidence that serotonin levels are linked to PMS. Remember, both mood and appetite centers are packed into the tiny hypothalamus. It is hoped that Redux might be able to alleviate PMS by keeping levels of serotonin in the brain high, elevating mood and decreasing appetite. Unfortunately, studies done with other serotonin-raising drugs have indicated they are not very successful in blocking the increased appetite PMS brings. This means that there are probably other effector pathways not linked to serotonin levels that account for the increase in appetite. Therefore, I do not recommend Redux for treating increased eating during PMS. The edema I described earlier should usually disappear within a few days of the completion of a woman's period. It is more of a nuisance than a health concern, but if the fluid persists, see your doctor. Some patients may require diuretics. The only recommendation I make to women who experience increased food intake during PMS is that they eat three big meals per day, with minimal snacking between meals. This discourages bingeing.

In my opinion, all weight-loss medications currently available, including Redux, will cause weight loss, on a substantial basis, for six to eight months. After that time, for some unknown reason, these medications cease to work for continuing weight loss. I believe that by this time, your new eating and evening exercise habits should be firmly established. The medication can then be used on an as-needed basis to keep weight off.

Incidentally, I encourage my patients to weigh themselves as often as twice a day. Surveillance takes work. Should one or two pounds creep back on, it's back to the Redux until they come back off. Initially, you used Redux to stop both your internal hunger signals and those emanating from any external cues. Now, your discipline and habits take over to put you in the driver's seat. You are free.

Remember in Chapter 2 that I promised you a chart that would show you emerging as the weight-loss winner? Here it is:

THE REDUX REVOLUTION	YOUR BODY'S RESPONSE
1. Phase I: Redux prescribed, along with the eating and exercise programs outlined in Chapters 5 and 6.	1. Appetite is suppressed; the gradual rate of weight loss tricks the brain into thinking that nothing is changing.
2. You practice meal reversal and nocturnal exercise over time.	2. Fat deposition is stopped. Your body is now in a weight-loss mode, and little muscle is lost.
3. Leptin levels fall slowly.	3. Neuropeptide Y is quiescent.
4. Phase II: Intermittent use of Redux; your new power of discipline is growing.	4. Cerebral cortex has stronger hold on appetite center of the hypothalamus.

5. Phase III: Occasional use of Redux only; appetite is controlled and weight loss is steady.	**5.** Insulin levels decrease over time, and hunger diminishes.
6. Your eating habits have now assumed those of a person having your goal weight!	**6.** Biochemically, you have altered your body's set point to match your new weight!

The health benefits that accompany weight loss are proportional to decreases in insulin levels and insulin resistance, which are directly related to the amount of fat lost. By losing weight in this scientifically "correct" fashion, you are switching your internal biochemical weight-gain mode to a weight-loss mode. The major health benefits you may attain depend upon your current health situation. If you have an obesity-related medical disorder, such as hypertension or diabetes, you will be able to control it better, either with or without medications. If you are disease-free, you lessen the risk of getting these diseases (see Chapter 10). And, of course, anyone who loses weight enjoys a better-looking body. You have done well for yourself, very well.

Yes, there is life after Redux. A healthy, fulfilling life!

DID YOU KNOW . . .

• One gram of alcohol contains seven calories, almost the same as fat at nine calories per gram.

• One martini contains the same amount of calories as 2½ slices of bread.

• Eating one meal a day may promote an enzyme that favors fat deposits: lipoprotein lipase.

• A goal of the U.S. government is to encourage at least

30% of all Americans to engage in regular physical activity by the year 2000 (currently, only 10% do so).

• Animals such as mice, dogs, and rats all become overweight by increasing the amount of fat in their diet.

• If you weigh 200 pounds, you expend 200 calories an hour typing 40 words a minute on an electric typewriter—this is only 70 calories less than walking at two miles an hour for an hour!

Chapter 8

The Phen/Fen Option

Thank you, Sarah Ferguson, Duchess of York. Recently, it was reported that "Fergie" lost 50 pounds while under a doctor's care. Her story was covered on the front page of the tabloids with dramatic before-and-after photos. Headlines read: "She looks smashing!" The papers reported that she had accomplished this through taking two weight-loss medications: phentermine and fenfluramine, the so-called phen/fen regimen. One of the tabloids, true to style, incorrectly reported that Fergie took amphetamines. Phentermine and fenfluramine are not amphetamines. The publicity had our phones ringing for weeks. My office manager, Betty, fielded numerous questions: "Does Dr. Levine use the same medications that Fergie took?" "I only want to lose 30 pounds—is it okay for me to take?" "I am much heavier than Fergie—will it work for me?"

Many of you have already heard of phen/fen, though it

surprises me that many others are still unaware of its existence despite an avalanche of media coverage. In 1994, ABC's *20/20* aired a flattering piece on the phen/fen regimen. This seemed to spark a phen/fen revival throughout the country. The two drugs made it to the covers of major news magazines and women's magazines and were featured in the *New York Times* and the *Wall Street Journal.* Television continues to carry an occasional story about these two medications. Right now, they are the rising stars of the pharmaceutical industry, and pharmacies can barely keep them on the shelves. This popularity stems from a tremendous grass-roots movement: Word is being spread by satisfied consumers. Even the Internet is abuzz with phen/fen!

"New" Weight-Loss Pills

Amazingly, these new weight-loss pills are not new! They predate Redux, as they were available in the 1970s, yet until recently they were largely ignored by the medical community and by the public as well. This was probably the result of poor timing. The 1970s were a time of optimism in the weight-loss field. The exercise boom was beginning, and many felt that jogging, bicycling, and swimming, coupled with "eating healthy," would help anyone lose weight. Also, this is the time when the amphetamine class of appetite suppressants, such as Dexedrine, became available (see Chapter 3). These drugs had such high side-effect profiles and were so grossly abused by so many that doctors tended to shy away from using them. In fact, doctors avoided using any medication to treat obesity, and the whole issue faded. To repeat: Phentermine and fenfluramine are not amphetamines, even though they

143

share some structural similarities with amphetamines. Phen/fen is effective and safe, and has little potential for abuse.

I find that the majority of people who take phen/fen actually have no idea how the drugs work. We will take a closer look at how these two drugs cause appetite suppression shortly. The two major misconceptions are:

• "They raise my metabolism." These drugs do not have any effect on metabolism. They work in the brain by suppressing appetite.

• "They burn fat." Phen/fen has no direct interaction with fat cells and does not burn fat.

Phen/fen is recommended for short-term use (about three months) by anyone over the age of 12 who is trying to lose weight. There are no specific guidelines at present as to who should use phen/fen. No one knows who will benefit from taking phen/fen and who won't. What prompted the sudden interest in phen/fen? The answer is: our nation's obesity problem.

A study done 12 years ago by Dr. Michael Weintraub of the University of Rochester Medical School tested phentermine and fenfluramine together. Prior to this time, each drug was tested by itself and results were mixed, at best. However, when the two drugs were combined, researchers were surprised to discover a powerful synergy that caused much greater weight loss than when either drug was used alone. There were fewer side effects in combining the drugs than would be expected, especially if you consider the side-effect profile of each drug individually. In fact, it appeared as if the side effects of one drug actually canceled the side effects of the other! Such a phenomenon is not often seen in clinical pharmacology.

The study was repeated by Dr. Weintraub in 1992 and appeared in the scientific journal *Clinical Pharmacology and Therapeutics*. In the second study, 121 patients, all with BMIs over 30 (130% to 180% of ideal body weight), were monitored in double-blind fashion for 34 weeks. A double-blind study, as you may remember from Chapter 3, is the gold standard for clinical evaluation of a medication. Patients were separated into two groups: those who took the phen/fen combination, and those who took a placebo medication. Both groups went through behavioral and nutritional counseling, as well as an exercise program. At 28 weeks, those who took phen/fen (15 mg phentermine and 60 mg fenfluramine a day) lost an average of 30 pounds. Those in the placebo group lost an average of 10 pounds. Later, when both groups took the drug intermittently for two years, some patients regained weight. However, the average weight loss for the phen/fen group after two years was still 22 pounds, and 19 pounds after three years. All of the patients who went off the drug regained their weight! The major side effects reported were dry mouth, diarrhea, fatigue, and nervousness.

As a result of this study, hundreds of physician-supervised weight-loss centers have sprung up across the country. They use phen/fen and have had, in general, good results with few major side effects.

Head to Head

The first question you might ask is: How does phen/fen stack up against Redux? I have used phen/fen on over 2,000 patients in the last few years. These patients have ranged in weight from 145 pounds to over 400 pounds. In my opinion, it is an excellent and safe regimen. Rather than compare the

145

two as competitors, we should look at them as complementing each other. Phen/fen stands on its own, and so does Redux. In medicine, no one drug works perfectly well in every clinical situation. Each patient requires custom therapeutic intervention. This is best illustrated by the pharmacological treatment of high blood pressure. A quick glance at the 1996 *Physicians' Desk Reference* shows that there are more than 100 antihypertensives (blood-pressure medications), alpha blockers, beta blockers, calcium channel blockers, angiotensin-converting enzyme inhibitors, and diuretics available today. Some of these medications work better in African-Americans, some work better in the elderly, and others perform best after a heart attack—different medications for different situations. No medical doctor would deny the need for them all! The same situation exists when treating obesity. Having another weapon against such a formidable foe is vital.

However, Redux has some important advantages:

• Redux may have greater efficacy—it may work better as an appetite suppressant. Studies comparing the two regimens are already in progress. Comparative analysis of the drugs is tricky, with many variables interfering with the proper interpretation of data. The real answer to the question of which drug is more effective may not even exist, but may actually depend on the biochemical makeup of the individual.

• Redux may be used, according to the FDA, for one year; phen/fen is allowed for use for three months. This difference has huge implications for long-term weight control. In fact, Redux is the only medication approved for both weight loss and maintenance, with the caution that the safety and effectiveness of Redux beyond one year have not been established.

• Redux is given two times a day. Phen/fen consists of two medications: Phentermine is taken once a day and fenfluramine is taken three times per day, for a total daily intake of four pills. In general, the more pills people must take in one day, the less likely they are to take all of them each day!

• Taking two different medications compounds the possibility of side effects.

Let's examine phentermine and fenfluramine individually.

Phentermine

Phentermine works on the appetite center in the hypothalamus. Unlike Redux, phentermine works to keep the levels of norepinephrine high in the brain. The name "norepinephrine" may be familiar to you. It's the precursor of the hormone epinephrine, which is commonly called adrenaline. Adrenaline is the "fight or flight" hormone. Having high levels of norepinephrine in the brain seems to dampen the appetite, causes people to eat faster, and lessens interest in food. Phentermine has no effect on serotonin, but it might affect another neurotransmitter called dopamine. Dopamine is a chemical found in the hypothalamus, as well as in other parts of the brain. It plays a role in our perception of reality and may act as a "gatekeeper" in controlling appetite. The higher our levels of dopamine, the more likely we are not to eat a great deal at any given time.

Its close relationship to adrenaline makes phentermine a central nervous system stimulant, and this is reflected in its side-effect profile:

• Dry mouth
• Insomnia—the inability to fall asleep, or remain asleep
• Tremor—"the shakes"

- Restlessness
- Nervousness
- Palpitations
- Rapid heartbeat
- Diarrhea
- Occasional increase or decrease in sexual drive (usually a decrease)

The chief side effects are dry mouth, which never causes patients to discontinue the medication, and insomnia, which can be corrected by lowering the dose or by taking phentermine first thing in the morning. Phentermine comes in both 15-mg and 30-mg strengths. Its listed side effects should not be confused with the side-effect profile of amphetamines. Phentermine's side effects are actually quite mild. Most people tolerate the drug well; few stop because of an adverse drug reaction. Occasionally, a patient will complain of a change in personality—either depression or, conversely, a type of euphoria.

M.G., a 60-year-old retired computer consultant, told me that he became quite manic at a Passover dinner, or Seder. He was taking 30 mg of phentermine. "I felt like I was a king at a feast. I was lecturing, insisting upon being the center of attention, and I was spouting an antireligious diatribe. All this in front of strangers. This wasn't me." While this behavior is not a typical side effect of the drug, we discussed lowering his dose. Incidentally, M.G.'s side-effect experience began after he had been on the phentermine for three months. This shows how any side effect can appear at any time in the course of treatment.

Then there is the euphoria, or "high" feeling, that is experienced by some patients. By my observation, this side effect occurs especially in females in their 30s to 50s who have

BMIs in the 25–27 range. It is interesting to note that even with steady weight loss, some of my patients feel cheated if they don't experience the same level of euphoria that their friends do! In my experience, this euphoria has not been a cause of abuse of the drug, and it fades in two to three weeks.

Phentermine does have some restrictions. It should not be used on children under 12. Alcohol should not be consumed with it, according to the manufacturer's label.

Contraindications (instances or conditions in which phentermine should not be prescribed) include:

- Advanced diseases of the arteries
- Symptomatic cardiac disease, such as angina
- Moderate to severe high blood pressure (hypertension)
- Glaucoma—increased pressure in the eye
- Hyperthyroidism—an overactive thyroid gland that has not been treated
- Any agitated state
- A history of drug abuse

It is ironic that hypertension should be on this list. While it is theoretically possible to elevate blood pressure with phentermine (as it is with over-the-counter and prescription decongestants), this rarely happens. After all, it is the obese patient with hypertension who needs to lose weight the most! The decision for a hypertension patient to take phentermine should be made on a case-by-case basis with the patient's doctor. The hyperthyroidism described here is the untreated type. Those patients who have had histories of overactive thyroid but who were treated for the condition should now be "euthyroid" (having normal thyroid function). They are good candidates for phen/fen if they are overweight. A quick blood test is all that is needed to check thyroid status. Glaucoma is a serious eye disease that is characterized by an increase of the internal pressure in the eye. Over time, this increase in pressure damages sensitive parts of the eye and causes blindness. If you do not know what your intraocular eye pressure is, you should have a quick and painless reading done at an ophthalmologist's office. If you already have glaucoma, check with your eye doctor before starting any weight-loss medication. As for drug abusers, phentermine does have a very slight potential for abuse, and I would not use it on this population.

There is another adverse drug interaction that deserves discussion. *Phentermine should not be used during, or 14 days after, the administration of monoamine oxidase inhibitors, or MAOs.* These are antidepressant drugs that include phenelzine sulfate (Nardil) and tranylcypromine (Parnate). If these drugs are taken with phentermine, blood pressure can rise to heart attack or stroke levels.

Fenfluramine

You may have noticed that this drug sounds a great deal like dexfenfluramine, or Redux. They are very closely related, as the chemical composition of Redux is a right-sided mirror image, or isomer, of fenfluramine. However, despite their common heritage, they are different. Because the appetite center of the brain is so sensitive, even slight alteration in the molecular structure of a medication can profoundly change its effect. Fenfluramine, like Redux, is a serotonin re-uptake inhibitor (see Chapter 3), but it is only 50% as potent as dexfenfluramine. It has a short half-life and so must be taken three

times a day, although it can be taken twice a day, or even
once in the evening.

Fenfluramine suppresses appetite and diminishes cravings
and binges between meals. It appears to have some effect on
women's premenstrual urges to eat, as well. Patients have told
me that they feel that the best thing about the drug is that it
takes away their preoccupation with food. It destroys what I
call the constant internal dialogue of asking yourself what's
for dinner when it's only breakfast time.

As far as side effects are concerned, fenfluramine has sed-
ative properties. (Remember, though, this effect is offset by
the stimulation of phentermine.) However, fatigue and depression are two side effects to watch out for with fenfluramine. Some patients complain of having dreams that are too
vivid. E.M., a 34-year-old physical therapist, complained that
she had a bad dream after her first dose of fenfluramine at
5:00 P.M. I checked the *Physicians' Desk Reference* and did not
find vivid dreams as one of the listed side effects for fenfluramine. I advised her to take it again the next evening. She
called the very next day, saying that the same problem had
recurred. I asked her to describe these dreams. She said, "I
am walking in a lush garden and I start to eat from a fruit tree.
I feel the juices from the fruit in my mouth, going into my
stomach, and I wake up with my heart beating very fast." I
asked her what was upsetting about her garden dream. She
replied, "You don't understand. It was so intensely real. I
never remember my dreams. These nights, I remember every
little detail. I thought my head was going to explode." She
stopped the fenfluramine and the dreams stopped. She is now
taking only phentermine and is doing well. These vivid
dreams are similar to those described by patients who took
LSD, the "tripping drug," back in the 1960s and 1970s. This

151

similarity comes as no surprise, as LSD has effects on serotonin levels.

The rest of the side-effect profile, as listed by the manufacturer, includes:

- Dry mouth
- Diarrhea
- Dizziness
- Insomnia
- Sweating
- Chills
- Increased urinary frequency
- Eye irritation
- Muscle pain
- Bad taste in mouth

The chief complaints voiced by patients are dry mouth, fatigue, depression, and diarrhea. These chief side effects are often mild and, similar to what we said previously about phentermine, they rarely cause cessation of the drug, but it happens. J.M., a teacher in her mid-40s, had to stop the drug. "I started to feel dizzy and nauseous, as if I were reexperiencing the bad morning sickness I had when I had my children. It starts one hour after I take the fenfluramine and lasts through the night." All of these side effects disappeared when the drug was stopped.

The major side effects of fenfluramine are similar to those of Redux and include primary pulmonary hypertension and short-term-memory changes. These are reviewed in our discussion of Redux's safety and side effects in Chapter 4. There is some indication that fenfluramine is less likely to cause PPH than dexfenfluramine is, but this has not been proved in studies. The same precautionary measures discussed in Chapter 4 for using Redux are implied for fenfluramine as well. The same precautions for drug interactions with Redux also apply to fenfluramine.

Sometimes having a certain side effect can be beneficial. For instance, in general, fenfluramine and dexfenfluramine induce a sleep state, or deepen a person's sleep. Before they begin treatment, many of my patients describe a peculiar habit of getting up in the middle of the night and eating. This can occur anywhere from the start of sleep until early morning! They describe it as being on "cruise control," a type of automatic behavior that runs itself. With fenfluramine working to help them sleep, they are much less likely to go on a midnight binge!

M.C., a 70-year-old pianist, was having trouble losing weight on the usual phen/fen regimen. What I had missed on the intake history of this patient was that she didn't eat large dinners, but she ate huge breakfasts. After a few weeks went by, and little weight was lost, we sat down again to discuss the timing of her meals. "I have a big breakfast every morning," she told me. When I asked what she eats, she said, "I just open the fridge and whatever is in there, I eat. Fish, meat, chicken, cheese, ice cream—anything and everything." I then asked what time she ate breakfast, "Oh, about 4:00 A.M." Then what? "I go back to sleep until 8:00 A.M., when I have a bagel and cream cheese." Isn't that two breakfasts? I asked. "No," she replied. "The 4:00-A.M. meal is breakfast, and the bagel with cream cheese is just a snack!" At this point, I realized that she was taking the fenfluramine too early, at 5:00 P.M. I changed her dose to 20 mg at 9:00 P.M. She slept better, stopped her 4:00-A.M. trips to the fridge, and has lost 70 pounds.

Tolerance to Phen/Fen

Tolerance to phen/fen develops quite commonly. Tolerance means that the more you take of a particular drug over time, the less the body responds to it, until the drug no longer works for you at all. Most people think of this as being immune to the drug, although this term is not medically correct. As time goes on, phen/fen can lose its effectiveness. You can almost sense it when you see the disappointment on the patients' faces before they tell you their story: "I think the drugs have stopped working, because I am getting hungry again." Or "I hear the food cabinets calling me again." This can be most disconcerting for a doctor, but it is one of the drawbacks to using phen/fen over time. This tolerance does not seem to occur with Redux, or at least it has not been documented clinically. However, with increased use, instances of tolerance will probably occur.

Fortunately, phen/fen can be restarted, after using two other drugs in its place. One is called diethylpropion (Tenuate) and the other is mazindol (Sanorex). Their actions and side-effect profiles are similar to those of phentermine. I use them to "buy time," until phen/fen can be restarted. Sometimes, these drugs give good weight-loss results by themselves and can be used until the patient stops losing weight or until an unpleasant side effect develops. The top dosage of diethylpropion is 75 mg, which can be given as one daily dose, or in three doses of 25 mg each, to be taken before meals. Mazindol's top dosage is 3 mg. It, too, can be given in one or two doses, taken before meals. This dosing flexibility allows doctors to customize a patient's regimen to use the least possible amount of drug to attain the most clinical benefit.

The Cost of Phen/Fen

The cost of the phen/fen regimen varies in different parts of the country. Some private insurance companies, as well as some HMOs, will cover at least part of your prescription. Unless you are certain that you are covered, obtain permission, in writing, from your insurance company for coverage before you start phen/fen. Also, because they are very "hot" drugs at the moment, there is great variation in pharmacy prices, which reflect local demand. Be sure to call different pharmacies to get the best prices. The two drugs together can cost between $65 and $95 per month.

Phen/fen has been used for over 25 years, and in general has an excellent safety record. For some patients, phen/fen will be a better option than Redux. Again, there are no head-to-head studies available yet. It is best to think of them as separate treatment options. However, in almost any clinical situation that Redux is used for in this book, phen/fen, or one of its component parts, can be tried. The same metabolism-enhancing guidelines should be followed that we discussed in Chapters 5 and 6. Of course, we must keep in mind that phen/fen is indicated for use only over a few months, and Redux can be used for up to one year.

Now you have the facts about both phen/fen and Redux. Deciding which regimen is best for you is an individual decision to be made by you and your doctor.

DID YOU KNOW . . .

• Americans spend $50 billion annually on weight loss, and this figure may double in the next five years!

• Doctors used to use thyroid extract to help patients lose weight, but it only caused muscle loss—not fat loss.

• Ephedrine, the chief component in Chinese herbs purported to cause weight loss, has caused seizures, heart attacks, and death.

• Chromium picolinate, an over-the-counter weight-loss medication, has caused cancer in mice at high doses.

• Over-the-counter diuretics, sometimes used for water loss, can cause life-threatening potassium loss.

• Phentermine is on the International Olympic Committee's list of banned drugs.

Chapter 9

Redux, Your Doctor, and You: Therapeutic Partners

Obesity is a private matter, yet Redux requires that a team approach be used. Since Redux is a potent medication that requires a prescription, you will have to go to your doctor to receive it. This begins what should be a working therapeutic relationship between you and your doctor. Redux brings new responsibilities to both parties.

Let's examine the doctor's side first. Traditionally, doctors have not been looked upon by patients as resources for weight loss. For the most part, doctors have had little training in weight loss, and the general consensus seems to be that patients fail so often that it's not worth the time or effort to engage patients in any weight-loss program. As a result, people who may have excellent doctor-patient relationships in other areas of health care have been seeking help from "alternative" sources—mail-order houses, health food stores, and diet centers—for weight loss.

Redux forces the medical community to rethink its approach to obesity—as if the state of our national health wouldn't be impetus enough! In light of new science regarding the obesity gene, leptin, and neuropeptide Y, in light of the FDA's approval of this viable medical weight-loss medication, doctors' offices will become the "weight-loss centers" of the next century. Redux will refocus doctors in the direction of learning more about Redux and perhaps expanding its use and application. It will encourage them to take an active role in patients' weight-loss concerns, just as they would in any other medical problem their patients might have.

Because millions of people suffer from obesity and its related health problems, weight-loss specialists cannot handle the load alone. This makes each doctor a potential weight-loss specialist. In order for this shift to occur, doctors must be willing to devote time to their weight-loss patients. The old cliché "Take two of these and call me in the morning" is not going to be enough. The responsibility doesn't end for doctors when they write the prescription for Redux; it is just beginning. Doctors must devise a follow-up plan. Obese patients need tremendous emotional support, and my advice to any physician or health professional reading this is: *In no way should Redux, or any weight-loss medication, be prescribed to patients unless you are prepared to counsel them and spend extra time with them.*

Now let's consider the patient's role. As a patient, you are essentially becoming your own round-the-clock weight-loss doctor, and you have responsibilities, too. First, you, too, must learn as much as you can about Redux, phen/fen, and other weight-loss medications. *The Redux™ Revolution* already puts you at the head of the class. Chances are, your physician has not had experience with Redux, as it is new to the United States, so you will almost be a "colleague" to your doctor in this area. It is up to you to initiate a therapeutic relationship with your doctor.

As a medical doctor, I can assure you that most doctors would welcome your partnership. Doctors, for whatever reasons they entered the field of medicine, have one universal characteristic: They all enjoy the feeling of being needed! In today's seemingly impersonal world of health care, the idea of establishing a therapeutic relationship, especially in an area as compelling as weight loss, would be very appealing to a doctor! If you feel that your doctor is not the right person to help you, find a doctor who is.

Another responsibility you have is to find out about cost and insurance coverage. Many HMOs and private insurance companies have special plans that cover treatment for weight loss. They are often not well advertised, so you must ask your agent directly. Keep in mind that when you ask whether your insurance covers for treatment of obesity, you may want to mention that you have an associated medical problem, like high blood pressure or diabetes, if that is in fact the case. Often, insurance companies will cover these secondary problems but will not cover obesity treatment alone. The cost of Redux may also be covered by your insurance. However, because it is a new medication in this country, you should obtain written verification that it will be covered. It would also be in your best interest to check Redux's price at different pharmacies, because there is often a large variation in price from store to store. It is to be hoped that Redux will be a catalyst in getting insurance companies to rethink their coverage of weight-loss treatment and related medications. Insurance companies stress the importance of preventive care and must recognize the importance of weight loss as preventive care. As you know from our discussion of "Syndrome X," losing weight prevents many health risks.

Medical weight loss should not be a privilege of the rich! In fact, most studies show that obesity is far more prevalent in the poorer communities of this country. This finding is in direct contrast to most other parts of the world, where the poor are thinner because of limited food supplies. Since diseases such as hypertension and diabetes are rampant in poorer communities, it is indeed fortunate that Redux is available to empower any local physician—in any office, hospital, or clinic—to help those who need it! Because weight loss is a key in improving health, and Redux is a key to losing weight, it is important that Redux be available to anyone who needs it, regardless of personal financial situation. For this reason, I believe that a cost-deferral plan should be implemented for those who need Redux but may not be able to afford it.

The first step in your weight-loss journey should be to make an appointment with your doctor to discuss what you want to accomplish with Redux and decide if your doctor is right for the job. Explain the ideas you have gained about eating and exercise through *The Redux™ Revolution*, review Redux's safety, and be prepared for the possibility that your doctor may not be as familiar with Redux as you are! That's fine; you can teach each other. Next, establish a follow-up schedule. There are currently no official follow-up guidelines for using any weight-loss medications, including Redux, so you and your doctor must create a follow-up schedule. Some patients require weekly visits, especially at the outset. Others require biweekly or monthly follow-ups. It is probably best for you to lean toward the conservative side in the beginning and schedule follow-up visits as often as possible. Also, ask your pharmacist to keep you informed of any new information released about Redux. Almost all pharmacies are computerized and receive up-to-the-minute electronic communiqués on all drugs that they stock.

Go Team!

So far, you have constructed a weight-loss team of three—you, Redux, and your doctor. You still need another one or two people to make your team complete. Think for a moment about the qualities you look for when putting together any team. You want people who exhibit an upbeat attitude, team spirit, and a strong work ethic, right? The same criteria should apply to the members of your weight-loss team. These additional facilitators can be friends, relatives, or coworkers. Their job is to help you handle any problem that may arise outside the scope of your visits to your doctor. The size of your facilitator group is not important, but the strength of each member's commitment to helping you is. You must tell each team member about how you and your doctor are planning your intake of Redux, about the evening eating deadline, and about the nocturnal exercise program. If possible, have team members attend one or two of your sessions with your doctor. This is a practice I strongly encourage.

Facilitators act as your personal cheerleaders. They should be people you can depend on for a kind word after a binge, a slip in discipline, or a moment of self-doubt. Why would you need the help of a weight-loss team? Because not only is the world an unfriendly place for the overweight, it is a downright hostile place for people trying to lose weight. The main obstacles take the form of what I call "the vicious triad."

The Vicious Triad

This triad consists of the top three reasons for weight-loss failure. These occur even on Redux, but they can often be anticipated and dealt with before they emerge. They are all interrelated, and each, on its own, can destroy a weight-loss effort. The three together virtually guarantee weight-loss failure. These threatening factors are:

1. Saboteurs
2. Bingeing
3. Depression

Saboteurs

These are the people who either consciously or unconsciously do not want you to succeed at weight loss. Believe it or not, they are usually people who are very close to you: a spouse, a brother or sister, a boyfriend, a parent, or a best friend. People who are trying to lose weight are extremely vulnerable, so these saboteurs often have a huge impact on them. In my practice, most of the saboteurs are spouses. You would think that most spouses would like their life partners to feel better about themselves and to be healthier as the result of weight loss. Yet I am constantly dismayed by attitudes that disprove this assumption, particularly those of husbands toward wives and boyfriends toward girlfriends. In my experience with over 2,000 patients, the majority of whom are women, only one husband has ever come into the office with his wife! *One!* Sabotage comes in many forms: lack of praise and encouragement, ignoring the particular needs of the dieter in terms of eating and exercise, offering inappropriate foods, and obvious jealousy over success. And these are just the ones I know about! What goes on at home must be tremendously stressful for my patients.

Saboteurs can also be friends or relatives, especially those who are overweight themselves. Weight-loss success seems to breed jealousy. I have seen countless patients with great attitudes lose weight, only to falter when a parent or friend says, "Sure, you're doing well now, but just wait. I lost 40 pounds last year and now I've gained back 50." When it comes to weight loss, prophecies of failure are almost always fulfilled. People who are trying to lose weight are particularly vulnerable because they are attempting something they have most likely failed at doing in the past. It's easy to throw them off their stride. I give patients several tips for coping with the saboteur dilemma:

• Transfer some of the self-doubt you have about succeeding at weight loss into the Redux capsule itself. Let Redux assume the brunt of the initial weight-loss effort, so you can invest your energies into feeling good about yourself. Weight loss should be a positive, pleasant experience.

• Identify the saboteurs before you start your weight-loss process. This will remove some of the power they have over you. In the end, sabotage is essentially a matter of control. If a person has no control over you, then what he or she says to you is only as important as you want it to be.

• Discuss this entire issue with your team. Perhaps the saboteur (though saboteurs are usually cowardly) will be willing to sit down with you and a member of your team and discuss more positive ways to help you.

• Seek professional counseling, especially if the saboteur is a spouse.

Bingeing

I can't tell you how many patients have sabotaged their own weight-loss efforts by bingeing. Even patients who have lost 40–50 pounds sometimes give in to temptation and go on a binge. From a doctor's perspective, I can tell you that this is the most frustrating aspect of treating the overweight. But hope is at hand in many cases. Here are some practical points on bingeing that relate to *The Redux™ Revolution*:

• There are people who have a separate disorder, known as binge eating disorder, or BED. This is a complicated syndrome and, like all eating disorders, often needs professional treatment. If you binge constantly, you should be evaluated as soon as possible. Redux does not work well against BED.

• Redux seems to be of particular value in combating ordinary binge eating. Remember that binge eating is related to mood changes, which are controlled in the hypothalamus next to the appetite centers. Serotonin probably plays a role in mood control as well. Low levels of serotonin can make you feel "down." Redux elevates the levels of serotonin around the clock, so you are less likely to binge.

• Bingeing around the time of menstruation is a normal phenomenon for many women, overweight or not.

• Often, bingeing is secondary to not eating regular meals. One of the main themes of *The Redux™ Revolution* is to eat "real" food at mealtime. Regular food will dampen any need to binge.

• Bingeing must not be followed by feelings of self-hatred.

Taking Redux will greatly reduce the amount of food eaten during a binge. If you continue to follow the evening time-table of eating and exercising outlined in Chapters 5 and 6, you will do fine. Remember, it is hard to gain weight rapidly. Don't forget that the body guards against rapid weight gain as well as weight loss. When you weigh yourself after a binge, the majority of the "new" weight will be from food not yet digested, or from water retention.

• Talk to a team member before a binge, if possible. It's not words of encouragement that will stop you, it's just the idea that you have identified a binge and are willing to do something about it. This is something you practice and get better at over time.

• Do not keep a large variety of high-calorie snack foods on hand. Few people binge on steaks, chicken, and tuna fish. It is usually some high-fat, high-carbohydrate food that is readily available for immediate consumption.

• Establish a plan. You should have a "compensating" option after a binge. This plan could include eating a "healthy" snack afterward to affirm that you know the difference between a healthy and an unhealthy snack. You may also perform some sort of exercise, making sure that you still follow the nighttime exercise guidelines outlined in Chapter 6. You should always have some sort of positive activity to follow a bingeing episode; this elevates serotonin levels and mood.

Speaking of moods, if there is one thing that will lead to weight-loss failure, it's depression.

The Diet Downer: Depression

Depression is a complicated issue, far beyond the scope of this book. Unfortunately, in my experience, depressed obese people do not lose weight. They can fool you into thinking they are doing well, but in the end they fail. If you are in a depressed state and don't care about yourself, for whatever reason, how can you care about something as demanding as losing weight? With the exception of psychiatrists, medical doctors are not well equipped to diagnose or treat depression. In the article "Prevalence of Repressive Symptoms in Primary Care" by William Zung, M.D., et al. in the 1993 *Journal of Family Practice*, it was estimated that nearly 20% of all patient visits were due to depression, while only 1% of patients cited depression as their reason for visiting the doctor. Patients generally listed somatic complaints, such as fatigue, headache, stomachache, and joint pain ahead of depression as their reason for seeing the doctor. The obvious implication here is that these are also symptoms of depression, not only missed by primary care physicians, but denied by the patients themselves.

Obesity is another clinical entity that can be added to this list. I estimate that seven out of every ten patients I see are depressed. I probably diagnose one or two out of ten on the first visit. These are the easy ones! Many people who are depressed deny that they are. Many doctors, myself included, are in denial as well. We feel that we can make a meaningful intervention in the patient's life if we ignore the depression and just treat the physical complaints. We are wrong! Overweight depressed people do not lose weight.

In my practice, my heart goes out to women whose husbands are unfaithful, to mothers who have suffered the loss of a child, to women whose children are disfigured or disabled, to single parents who are struggling to survive financially. The depth of their pain is matched only by their courage to live life as normally as possible. How can weight loss matter to these people? Redux is strong medicine, but not strong enough to overcome a patient's depression.

Merely being overweight is not the cause of my patients' depression, in most cases. This is a misconception thin people often have. However, it is true that obesity can compound a depression that is already present. The negative social stigma associated with being overweight may help to explain this phenomenon. A recent study mentioned in the June 1996 issue of *Allure* brings this point home. Two researchers from St. Edward's University in Austin, Texas, placed two different phony personal ads in local newspapers. One described the advertiser as being 50 pounds overweight. The other claimed to be an ex-addict, recovering for the last 11 months. The ex-addict received 30 queries, while the overweight woman received only eight! The respondents would rather date an ex-addict than an overweight person!

If Redux isn't the answer for depression, then what is? I believe the first step is "coming out of the pantry." You must admit both of these things to yourself: I am overweight and I am depressed. Next, you should treat the depression first. As I said before—and I want to be very clear about it—depressed overweight people do not lose weight. By treatment, I mean going to a psychiatrist or psychologist and perhaps using one of the newer class of "selective serotonin re-uptake inhibitor" antidepressants, such as fluoxetine (Prozac). Once you feel better about yourself, Redux is waiting for you.

Few people actually view themselves as depressed. The symptoms of depression can be subtle. Here is a sample of some of the questions I ask patients to determine if depression is contributing to the way they are feeling:

- Do you feel distant from other people?
- Does your weight gain make you feel less attractive?
- Do you enjoy your work?
- Do you often lack energy?
- Have you contemplated "bad" things happening to you?
- Do you have increased headaches, stomachaches, or joint pains?
- Do you feel distant from your family?
- Does your family support your weight loss?
- Have you been sleeping too much lately?
- Do you have trouble falling asleep?
- Has your social or sex life changed since you gained weight?

It's important that both patients and doctors become more aware of the symptoms of depression, so it can be therapeutically addressed and patients can move on to weight-loss success. Having your team in place can ensure that, together, you're doing all you can to succeed in reaching your weight-loss goals.

DID YOU KNOW . . .

- Some studies suggest that follow-up visits, by themselves, cause weight loss, as opposed to weight-loss medications.
- Twiggy, who started the "thin" model craze in the 1960s, was 5'7" and weighed 92 pounds.
- The *Venus of Willendorf*, a Paleolithic stone figure and one of the earliest known renderings of the human form, is extremely obese.

• There are an estimated 20 million Americans who suffer chronic depression.

• There is a form of depression called "smiling" depression, in which the patient displays outward cheerfulness.

• Depression is more common in women.

Chapter 10

Health 2000: Saved by the Millennium?

11:59, December 31, 1999. In just one second, with the blessing of Dick Clark, the new millennium will arrive. You ready your glass of champagne to toast the next thousand years. Are you at your peak level of health today, or are you going to start pursuing better health with that toast? This is a question you may ask yourself, but the American government wants to know the answer as well. In 1987, a "think tank" was assembled to discuss the health issues that affect our nation most. Utilizing the expert advice of nearly 10,000 individuals, this national health consortium established an ambitious goal: to provide a blueprint to show the way to a healthier America by the year 2000. The result of their work was the book *Healthy People 2000*, published in 1991. It is probably available at your local library. Among the health concerns that are stressed in the book as affecting our national health are obesity and three of its closely related disorders: high blood pressure, adult-onset diabetes, and uterine cancer. *Healthy People 2000* clearly states that we, as a nation, can do a better job of preventing, diagnosing, and controlling these diseases. As a result, we, as Americans, can extend the amount of time that we live healthy lives.

Better overall health now and in the future can be attained through weight loss, and as stated in Chapter 1, even a small amount of weight loss can help. Nature must have been in one of her better moods when she decided, eons ago, that we would have the power to control these diseases and live longer through weight loss. In helping us tackle these three illnesses, Redux may have its most powerful impact on our overall health. This benefit can only begin to be a reality when we reexamine our collective definition of obesity as a mere cosmetic problem and acknowledge the true dangers that accompany it. Too often, people feel that the problems related to obesity only affect other people. In reality, the "other people" are essentially us: obesity, hypertension, and uterine cancer affect 80 to 100 million people!

The Redux™ *Revolution* proposes that we take a more aggressive role in safeguarding our own health. For every disease there are two paths to follow. The first is passive—accepting the diagnosis of hypertension or diabetes, taking medication for life, and playing Russian roulette with side effects. In essence, you are a victim of either the disease or the effects of the medication, and you may eventually succumb to illness despite the medication.

The other path is active. You know that weight loss is the key in controlling hypertension and diabetes and in helping prevent uterine cancer if you are overweight. You now have Redux and a plan to combat these ailments! Follow this plan, and you can make immediate biochemical changes in your body that favor your health! Let's take a closer look at the diseases we've been addressing.

Hypertension

A staggering 45 million people in this country have high blood pressure. This number translates to one out of every five Caucasian adults. Hypertension is rampant in the African-American population, where its incidence is double that among the white population. It occurs with equal frequency in men and women, and it can even affect children. Unbelievably, there are millions of Americans who still don't know what their blood pressure is. Do you? You should, because it's known as the "silent killer." All too often, the first symptom is also the patient's last. Sudden death from heart attack or stroke can occur in people with high blood pressure. Amazingly, it is estimated that even among the millions of people on blood pressure medication, only 35% have their hypertension under control.

Arbitrarily defined as a blood pressure reading above 140/90, hypertension is the medical term for high blood pressure. The higher number is called the systolic pressure and the lower number is the diastolic. Often, patients are under the misconception that only one number "counts" in relation to increased risk of cardiovascular disease with high blood pressure. They posit that a blood pressure of 180/90 is nothing to worry about because the lower number, the diastolic pressure, is normal. Sometimes, patients with a blood pressure of 140/110 believe they are in good shape because only the bottom number, the diastolic pressure, is elevated. In reality, both numbers are important, though the upper number is perhaps more important in predicting future cardiovascular risk. The higher a patient's systolic pressure, the more likely it is that cardiac disease will be a factor in that individual's future. Basically, the systolic pressure is the pressure exerted against the arterial walls when the heart is pumping the blood through the body. The lower number, or diastolic pressure, is the pressure that the blood exerts on the arterial walls when the heart is in a relaxed mode, between beats.

The function of the arteries is to supply nutrient- and oxygen-rich blood to the organs. In order for this to occur, arteries themselves must be elastic—they must flex as more blood flows through them, and relax when less blood flows. This is a normal phenomenon. In someone with hypertension, the increased pressure characteristic of hypertension is stressing the inside walls of the arteries, destroying their elasticity. Should this same person have atherosclerosis, or hardening of the arteries, especially in the context of "Syndrome X" (see Chapter 2), then he or she would also have high insulin levels, high cholesterol, and abnormal clotting factors. Now things literally get "sticky." High levels of cholesterol and insulin attract platelets in the blood to form plaques of fatty deposits that adhere to arterial walls, narrowing them. This scenario can happen to anyone, but it seems to be accelerated in the obese who have Syndrome X. Ultimately, this combination of increased blood pressure, hardening of the arteries, and plaques on the arterial walls leads to a greatly diminished blood flow in the affected area. This can lead to several health hazards, depending on the affected area. These hazards include heart attack (blockage in coronary arteries), decreased vision or blindness (blockage in the vessels of the eyes), kidney failure (blockage in the vessels that lead to the kidneys), and stroke (blockage in the vessels in and leading to the brain).

The higher the blood pressure, the greater the risk for these problems, and the worse the prognosis for recovery. The exact cause of hypertension is unknown; however, many cases of hypertension are due in great part to being overweight. Fortunately, blood pressure can be lowered effectively with even mild weight loss, and Redux can be used to help this weight loss. Please keep in mind that caution must be exercised when using Redux in patients with severe, uncontrolled hypertension. The contraindications for Redux are listed in Chapter 4.

There are more than 100 different medications used to treat hypertension, including alpha blockers, beta blockers, calcium channel blockers, and diuretics. All work well, but all are fraught with side effects. Often, neither doctors nor patients are thinking about the treatment option that gives the patient the best chance to walk down the assertive path. This treatment option includes weight-loss medications like Redux.

There are many studies that show that Redux not only can lower blood pressure through weight loss but may actually have a beneficial effect on blood pressure independent of a change in weight! One of these studies, done in Belgium, entitled "Effect of Dexfenfluramine Treatment on Body Weight, Blood Pressure, and Noradrenergic Activity in Obese Hypertensive Patients," by Dr. J. Kolanowski et al., was published in 1992 in the *European Journal of Clinical Pharmacology*. These researchers found that Redux (dexfenfluramine) caused an average of 12 pounds of weight loss after three months of use in a group of 15 "borderline" hypertensive patients. The study defined "borderline" hypertensivity as anyone with blood pressure slightly over 140/90. None was on blood pressure medication. Not only did the blood pressure normalize, but Redux lowered both catecholamines and insulin—body chemicals that are assumed to play a major role in hypertension—at a rate greater than that expected from weight loss alone. Catecholamines, such as epinephrine and norepinephrine, are hormones secreted in the adrenal glands, above the kidneys. These two substances are presumed to promote high blood pressure by causing constriction of the arteries.

In short, Redux's benefit for hypertension goes beyond weight loss. Also, Redux has been shown to lower other risk factors for heart disease, such as clotting factors and elevated cholesterol.

Here is an example of a woman, a "Syndrome X-er," who chose to take the second path and do something about her hypertension. S.M., a 41-year-old mother of two, was diagnosed with hypertension three months earlier. Her blood pressure was 160/100. Her labwork and EKG were normal. Her doctor started her on a calcium channel blocker. Her blood pressure went down to 130/90, but she developed edema (fluid) in her legs. Her doctor switched her to a beta blocker. This medication made her tired. She came into my office when her insurance switched to an HMO in which her original doctor was not a member. When I first saw her, her weight was 141 pounds at 5'1" and her blood pressure was 160/100. Although we might not think of her as obese, she did have a BMI (see Chapter 1) of 27. She would be a candidate for Redux because she also had hypertension, a complication of obesity. She was started on the phen/fen regimen and was directed to follow the evening diet and exercise regimen outlined in Chapters 5 and 6. She lost 12 pounds in two months and her blood pressure is now 130/80, without medication! She no longer takes phen/fen, but she continues the evening diet and exercise regimen.

This case illustrates how modest weight loss, aided by

weight-loss medications, allowed this woman to change her health outlook. She chose the active second path, and now she is reaping the health rewards!

Adult-Onset Diabetes

Adult-onset diabetes (Type II) is currently a national health crisis. Thirteen million Americans have this disease, and 40,000 new cases are diagnosed every month—that's one every 60 seconds! Nine out of ten adult-onset diabetics are overweight. Please, do not confuse this disease with the childhood illness of diabetes (Type I). There are currently approximately 5 million Americans who have adult-onset diabetes and do not know it—a situation similar to that of hypertension. Adult-onset diabetes is like obesity in that it is a highly genetic disease; childhood diabetes is not. If you are not aware of the symptoms of diabetes, they include:

- Fatigue
- Increased thirst
- Increased urination
- Nighttime urination
- Blurred vision
- Urinary tract infections that are difficult to treat
- Any unusual skin infections

If you have any of these symptoms, see your doctor.

Diabetes is a frequent cause of heart disease, sudden death, kidney failure, blindness, sexual impotence, nervous-system damage, and circulation problems that may lead to foot ulcer and toe or foot amputations. Amazingly, just as with hypertension, moderate weight loss can control diabetes. With dramatic weight loss, many cases of diabetes can even be cured.

However, there is a snag. Virtually all patients who are obese and who have diabetes, or who have first-degree relatives with diabetes and are prime candidates for a prevention program, have insulin resistance, which we discussed in Chapter 2. These people are always hungry because their insulin levels are high. Few doctors would disagree that the odds of an overweight diabetic losing weight are dismal. This situation could change with Redux.

Not only has Redux been shown to cause the weight loss that diabetics so desperately need, but it may have a beneficial effect in lowering blood sugar as well! It is unclear how Redux accomplishes this, but it probably involves lessening the liver's capacity to release sugar in the blood. The main point here for diabetics and hypertensives is: You *must* do all you can to lose weight. You *must* make yourselves go down that second path, and Redux may help.

Here is a story of two men, unknown to each other, born in the same year of 1919. Both men played college football: one on the West Coast in Division I, the other on the East Coast in Division III. Both men received offers from professional football teams after college, and both chose careers outside football. The Division I player went on to have a Hall of Fame baseball career. He developed adult-onset diabetes. After his retirement, his eyesight became so poor that, to the dismay of his former teammates, he could barely recognize his old friends at team reunions. He continued to put on weight, and in 1972, at the age of 53, he died of a heart attack. His name is Jackie Robinson, and he is a hero to many, known as the man who broke the color barrier in baseball.

The other man, S.L., was rushed to the emergency room of his local hospital in 1976. His blood sugar was 480, four times the normal level. It came as a complete surprise to him that he was in a high-risk group for diabetes—he weighed 35 pounds over his playing weight of 215 pounds, and the majority of his extra weight was around his midsection. His mother, also a diabetic, had died suddenly of a stroke at age 63. (I hope by this point you are reminded of "apples" and "Syndrome X," which we discussed in earlier chapters. If so, good for you—you're learning!) S.L. was treated with intravenous fluids, kept overnight for observation, and discharged in the morning with a diabetic "pill" to control his blood sugar. He was told to exercise, to follow a 1,500-calorie American Diabetes Association diet, and to follow up regularly with his doctor. Today, 80 pounds lighter, S.L. is a vigorous, trim man of 77. He is a very active accountant, and a good one. Amazingly, that emergency-room visit was his last contact with diabetes. He cured himself through weight loss without medication. He overcame his own insulin resistance, probably by applying to his weight-loss regimen the discipline he had learned as an athlete.

How do I know this case so well? S.L. is my father, Sol Levine, and I am very proud of him. He chose to take the active path, took charge of his medical problem, and cured himself of diabetes. My father accomplished this before the Redux Revolution. However, Redux can give almost anyone with Type II diabetes a chance to do what my father did: choose their own path for health!

Uterine Cancer

Uterine cancer is the genital cancer most frequently seen in women. It is the third most common cancer in women, after breast and colon cancer. Its peak incidence is in the 50-to-60-year-old age group. Risk factors for uterine cancer are:

1. Obesity
2. The use of female hormones
3. Age greater than 40
4. Infertility
5. Women who have never ovulated

In postmenopausal women, the chief symptom of uterine cancer is abnormal uterine bleeding. One-third of all cases of women with abnormal uterine bleeding after menopause result in a diagnosis of uterine cancer.

According to Dr. Bruce Meller, attending gynecologist at Beth Israel Hospital in New York City, "There are 30,000 new cases of this type of cancer per year. Obesity is one of the proposed factors of its cause. Excess body fat interferes with the metabolism of various female hormones that act to counterbalance the effects of estrogen on the female body. This keeps the level of estrogens higher than normal, and this constant unopposed action of estrogen on the uterus can cause cancer."

To lessen her risk of uterine cancer, an overweight woman can follow the plan outlined in *The Redux™ Revolution* and lose weight. Although obesity is not the only risk factor for uterine cancer, it is a major one. This is one form of cancer we know can be prevented in great measure. It is up to you!

Other Health Problems of Obese Women

Other problems unique to women that are related to obesity include:

1. Menstrual problems—ranging from abnormal bleeding episodes to amenorrhea, the lack of menstruation
2. Fertility disorders
3. Higher incidence of cesarean births
4. Higher incidence of gestational diabetes (a form of diabetes that occurs during pregnancy)
5. Higher incidence of spontaneous abortion

Moreover, a study by M. M. Werler, recently published in the *Journal of the American Medical Association,* painted a bleak possibility for overweight mothers-to-be. Women who weigh more than 242 pounds prior to pregnancy have a four-times-greater risk of having a child with spina bifida, an incomplete closure of the spinal column, which can result in paralysis and loss of brain matter. Approximately 2,500 babies are born with spina bifida each year. Women who weigh between 176 and 195 pounds prior to pregnancy have a two-times-greater risk of having a child with spina bifida. Using Redux to cause weight loss in an overweight woman contemplating pregnancy can now not only benefit the potential mother, but also prevent disease in the baby-to-be!

The scope of medical problems associated with obesity go far beyond hypertension, diabetes, and female reproductive problems. These, too, can be treated most effectively with Redux and weight loss. They include:

• Varicose veins
• Blood clots in the extremities
• Gout
• Osteoarthritis
• Foot pain
• Fatty infiltration of the liver
• Gallbladder disease

• Hernias
• Skin infection in skin-fold areas

Live Longer with Weight Loss

Everyone wants to live longer! Because no one is certain about what happens on "the other side," we want to stay on "this side" for as long as we can. Does weight loss have any effect on longevity? We already learned in Chapter 1 that the morbidly obese are candidates for sudden death. We also learned that being 20% over ideal body weight can make you prone to cardiovascular disease, hypertension, and diabetes. But what is the "perfect weight"—the one that allows for the longest life?

Thanks to a huge nationwide study, there is an answer! Researchers at Harvard Medical School have conducted a 16-year study, the Nurses' Health Study, which has looked at the relationship of body weight and mortality among women. The study took place from 1976 to 1992, and 115,000 registered nurses completed questionnaires for it. In the case of each woman, BMI (Body Mass Index; see Chapter 1), waist/hip ratio, and comparative body weight were analyzed at prescribed intervals beginning at age 18. The results revealed four important points:

• A weight gain of 22 pounds or more after the age of 18 is associated with increased mortality in middle adulthood.
• A BMI above 27 increases mortality.
• A weight gain of 11 to 18 pounds in adult life resulted in a higher risk of heart disease.
• Moderately overweight women are at risk for nonfatal heart attack, gallbladder disease, hypertension, and diabetes.

Are you ready to take the second path toward good health—the one of action? Or are you going to remain passive about assuming control over your health? The overwhelming message from all the latest research is clear: Modest weight loss can yield enormous long-term health benefits. By taking advantage of the Redux Revolution, you can live a longer, healthier life.

With Redux, you can become thinner and healthier in this millennium! Go for it!

DID YOU KNOW . . .

• Every 60 seconds, another person is diagnosed with adult-onset diabetes.

• By the year 2000, close to 20 million people in the United States will be diagnosed as having adult-onset diabetes.

• Over the past few years, 10% of all pregnant women in the United States have been obese prior to pregnancy.

• Physicians receive 100 million patient visits per year due to hypertension.

• About 85,000 diabetics each year receive lower-extremity amputations.

• Obese pregnant women have a higher incidence of having a child born with Down syndrome.

Chapter 11

Redux and Smoking: Quit Now and Lose Weight!

My uncle Dr. Harold Levine, a man I respected both personally and professionally, had eyes that could not only talk—they could scream! I witnessed those eyes respond to many things, but the topic that invariably drew the biggest reaction was smoking. My uncle had a personal crusade against smoking and would do almost anything to get people to quit, including accosting smokers on the street and handing them antismoking literature. His success in getting many people to quit was a testament to his persistence. It also demonstrates the importance of counseling and of a health professional's taking a personal interest in the patient's outcome.

Keep in mind, these were the days before any medical treatment for nicotine withdrawal was available. The patients who quit did so virtually on their own, "cold turkey." While this approach may seem a bit harsh to some, for Dr. Harold

Levine, it was a way of life—literally. During the 1970s, this world-renowned expert on lung disease was Chief of Pulmonary Medicine at the VA Hospital in Chicago and Professor of Medicine at the Stritch College of Medicine of Loyola University, Chicago. A pioneer in the war on tobacco, he served on President Johnson's antismoking committee. This crusade against smoking was fueled by one startling fact: One out of every two smokers will die prematurely from a smoking-related disease.

I share my uncle's antismoking passion and have made efforts to encourage and enable people to quit, including my ten-step "Quit and Lose" program outlined in this chapter. As I think about the chilling realities of the harmful effects of smoking, I am reminded of a commercial I saw several years back. In it, a famous actor who was suffering from lung cancer—the result of many years of heavy smoking—was leaving his final legacy: a message against smoking. His words: "When you see this commercial, I will be dead. This happened because of smoking. If you smoke, quit. If you don't smoke, don't start." The man delivering this message was none other than the late Yul Brynner, who died of lung cancer. Why, then, don't people listen to the facts? Why didn't people listen to Yul? Why don't smokers just quit?

The fact is, most have tried. Unfortunately, 90% of all smokers have tried to quit at one point or another, but without much success. There are two chief reasons for this dismal rate:

- The difficulty of overcoming the effects of withdrawal from nicotine addiction
- The fear of gaining weight

Redux for Your Lungs!

To address the first issue, medical science has introduced nicotine gums, nicotine patches, and more recently nicotine nasal spray. These products reduce the withdrawal symptoms that many smokers fear. They work extremely well when used in conjunction with a support program, which is discussed later in this chapter.

Now science has come up with an effective way to address the second issue and prevent the weight gain. Redux or phen/fen can now be used with the nicotine-withdrawal medications, so that overweight smokers can quit and lose weight at the same time! This novel concept is a surprisingly simple one, and involves following the ten-step program below.

While there is no official indication from the manufacturers of these drugs for using the medications in this fashion, they do work. There are now many studies in worldwide medical literature that have shown success using this combined approach. Because smoking cessation is so important, this method should be attempted by any smoker who is overweight and wants to quit. The rationale behind using the medication is simple. Smoking increases the body's metabolic rate. So when a person quits smoking, the metabolic rate drops, increasing appetite and causing weight gain. This is a common phenomenon experienced by numerous ex-smokers—especially during the first six to 12 months after smoking cessation. Many have expressed the opinion that quitting "isn't even worth it" because the ensuing weight gain is so depressing. Using the drugs eliminates the increase in appetite and actually makes it possible to lose, not gain, weight after smoking cessation.

Our First Success

The first hint I had that this plan could be feasible came from L.F., an accounts manager. A longtime smoker, weighing 208 pounds, she came to my office for weight loss only, with no intention of quitting smoking. She was started on the phen/ fen program and after four weeks had lost nine pounds and had gained a great deal of self-esteem. At this point, she asked me if I could help her quit smoking once she reached her "goal" weight. Thinking she might change her mind if I didn't act quickly, I asked, "Why not start now and quit with the nicotine patch?"

She replied, "I want to concentrate on one vice at a time. It's tough enough to lose weight without any distractions. I want to concentrate on the weight loss."

She had a valid point, but I took a chance and repeated my suggestion that she try the nicotine patch while continuing the phen/fen regimen. We agreed that if she had any problems with the weight loss, we would stop the patch. I wasn't aware of any drug interaction between phen/fen and the nicotine patch, so I knew it was safe. Because patients have depressed metabolic rates for six months to a year after quitting smoking, the plan was to continue the phen/fen regimen on an as-needed basis during this period, even if her weight-loss goal had been met. In this way, the increase in her appetite after smoking cessation would still be controlled and would not undo her successful weight loss.

It worked! L.F. quit smoking and continued to lose weight, actually stopping the patch after only two months. She has since lost 55 pounds, and after 14 months, not only has she kept the weight off, but she has not smoked, either. She looks 15 years younger and radiates health when she stops in to say hello. Defying traditional medical logic, L.F. quit smoking and lost weight! The combination of the nicotine patch and the phen/fen works! A first case for me, but success must begin somewhere.

Reality Bytes

In 1995 alone, 400,000 Americans died from smoking-related diseases such as emphysema, lung cancer, and heart disease. The same sad statistics occur year in and year out. In 1982, as a medical intern at Mt. Carmel Mercy Hospital in Detroit, I was involved in the care of a 29-year-old woman admitted for the workup following an abnormal chest X ray. She had been a smoker for six years and had had a recurring cough for about a month. Frightened, she asked me if it could be cancer. With my lack of experience and considering her age and relatively short smoking history, I told her that I doubted it. I was wrong—dead wrong! In just two short months she died, leaving behind a husband and two small children.

A few weeks later, I approached one of the staff oncologists (a doctor specializing in the treatment of cancer) and asked him, "Isn't it true that you have to smoke thousands of cigarettes to contract lung cancer, and isn't it a disease of people in their 50s and 60s?"

His response shocked me. "No," he said. "In fact, theoretically, one cigarette alone can cause cancer, because it only takes one tiny cigarette-induced mutation to one tiny cell to start the cancer process." He then added, "Incidentally, lung cancer rates in women have risen 500% since the 1960s!"

Each day, 3,000 adolescents become addicted to nicotine and become regular smokers. That's a million a year! One of those kids could be your son, daughter, grandchild, niece, or nephew. Keep this figure in mind—the tobacco industry certainly does! Each year tobacco companies sell $1 billion worth of cigarettes to 3 million adolescents. One of the biggest fears of these adolescents—one that prevents them from quitting—is the threat of weight gain. This concern must not be minimized and has much to do with distorted body image and peer pressure. Parents and physicians must take an active stand, not just to implore kids to quit. The specific need that these teenagers have not to gain weight must be addressed. They must be made aware that there is a way to stop smoking without gaining weight.

The Ten-Step "Quit and Lose" Program

The time to quit is now. Here is my ten-step method of combining anti-nicotine and weight-loss medications so you can quit and lose weight at the same time.

Step 1. Commit to the program. Each person has his or her own reasons for wanting to quit, ranging from "I don't want to get cancer" to "My hair smells" or even "My husband/wife hates it." Much more important than having a reason to quit, however, is committing to a structured approach that incorporates support, like this one. Studies show that trying to do it by yourself, even using the nicotine patch, does not work.

NOTE: A great reason to quit is that children who live in the household of smokers are prone to ear infections, bronchitis, and asthma. Do it for them, but commit to it for yourself!

Step 2. Find a supportive doctor who has experience with smoking cessation and weight loss. Again, you can use the extra support. It's not going to happen by doing it yourself. NOTE: You may have to introduce this new concept of quitting smoking while losing weight to your doctor after reading *The Redux™ Revolution.*

Step 3. Discuss treatment options with your doctor. This seems self-explanatory, but it is actually the most important step, and one often neglected by both doctor and patient. You must learn your anti-withdrawal options. There are four different nicotine patches currently available, some of which are now available over the counter:

• Habitrol
• Nicoderm
• Nicotrol 16
• Prostep

These patches are applied to the skin, and each patch is kept there for 24 hours. Because there are four different kinds, you have considerable dosing flexibility, and you and your doctor can switch brands if one doesn't work. The basic idea behind the patch is to deliver decreasing doses of nicotine to the patient through the skin. This allows the patient to avoid the unpleasant nicotine withdrawal symptoms that can occur after smoking cessation and that can lead to smoking again. The length of time the patient uses the patch depends on the individual. Some patients may use it for up to a year, or even longer, before they feel comfortable without it. The same applies to the use of nicotine gum. These gums work by the same principle as the patch. They come in 2-mg and 4-mg strengths and can be used for maintenance.

The Federal Drug Administration recently approved Nicotrol as the first nicotine nasal spray. It is supposed to be as effective as the gums or patches, but according to its manufacturer, McNeil Pharmaceutical, it relieves nicotine cravings even faster. Since this is a brand-new medication, I would consider it a "second line" in our plan, until there are more clinical trials to give evidence that the spray works as well as the patch and gum.

NOTE: Doctors' offices and pharmacies have a great deal of information available on these nicotine medications. Ask for it and read it! Some manufacturers even have 24-hour phone support services, while others provide audio tapes. Remember that the more support you have from as many sources as possible, the better your chances of success.

NOTE: Many patients can quit without the patch, depending on the level of nicotine addiction. If you feel you are one of these people, skip to Step 9.

Step 4. Start Redux or phen/fen with the same metabolism-raising plan outlined in Chapters 5 and 6.

To reiterate, there are no known interactions between Redux or phen/fen and the nicotine patch or gum. However, caution should be exercised when using the nicotine patch with phentermine. Because they both have stimulant-like side effects, they can make you edgy or wakeful. Other possible side effects include skin irritation at the site of the application of the patch, unpleasant dreams, and stimulation. This last side effect occurs most often when the doctor initially prescribes too strong a dose.

Step 5. Lose the first five to ten pounds over two to three weeks, depending on your initial weight. Obviously, the less you weigh, the more time you will need to lose the initial weight. This initial weight loss will put your body in a "weight-loss mode." It will also give you a good psychological boost to continue.

NOTE: *Do not start any nicotine preparation until this initial weight is lost.* This is a trick of the trade.

Step 6. Start the nicotine gum or patch *only after completing Step 5.* If you have been a heavy smoker (more than a pack a day over twenty years or the equivalent) and have tried to quit many times in the past, you may need more help. This is especially true if you have been unable to quit using the patch or the gum only. In this case, your doctor can prescribe the nicotine gum and the nicotine patch, to be taken simultaneously. Be aware that the possibility of additive side effects is present—that is, you can increase the number of side effects by using the patch and gum together. However, most patients have no problem with this regimen.

Step 7. Follow up with your doctor every two to four weeks for the first six months. Remember, getting support is just as important as taking the medications. Also, you should be monitored for any unforeseen side effects, such as abnormal dreams or occasional nighttime binge eating. This follow-up is of the utmost importance. It is assumed that the same doctor will be treating you for weight loss and smoking cessation, so a separate visit for the two is not necessary.

NOTE: If you notice that you are having difficulties handling both weight loss and smoking cessation for *any* reason, do not wait for your scheduled appointment—see the doctor as soon as possible. An immediate relapse is often difficult to treat.

Step 8. Working with your doctor, taper the dose of your nicotine preparation. Keep in mind that the timing of this step varies with the individual. Some patients taper and stop their nicotine preparation almost immediately, while others continue for many months. Some people may still have the urge to smoke. You must inform your doctor if you start to smoke again, because the dosage of the patch or gum must be reduced.

Step 9. Continue the weight-loss pills on an as-needed basis for at least six to 12 months from the day you quit, even after weight-loss goals have been met. This is to guard against the appetite increase that inevitably follows smoking cessation. These months are a very vulnerable time, so it is crucial that you follow up with your doctor.

Step 10. Stop the weight-loss pills after six to 12 months, if your weight-loss goals have been met.

This vulnerable time after smoking cessation varies with the individual, depending on the length of time and the amount (per day) of smoking. After this time, use the pills on the as-needed basis previously prescribed for nonsmokers.

Deborah's Story

The ten-step program outlined above includes suggested guidelines only. They may be modified to meet the individual needs of patients. For instance, Deborah, a 43-year-old marketing analyst, wanted to lose weight and quit smoking together. She loved aerobic dancing, but at 5'3" and 175 pounds, she found her legs "too heavy to move," and her "wind was gone." She was started on phen/fen and given the nicotine patch. However, within 24 hours, Deborah was having problems with palpitations and feelings of nervousness. I lowered the dosage of her patch, but she still had problems with palpitations. Her pulse was at 88, whereas a normal pulse for her was 64. Ultimately, we stopped the patch altogether and Deborah quit "cold turkey." However, it seems that the mild stimulant properties of phentermine countered the lack of nicotine in her system, and so her smoking cessation and weight loss continued! After five months, Deborah has stayed away from cigarettes, and her weight is down to 134 pounds. Now when Deborah comes into the office wearing her aerobic tights, she doesn't walk—she dances! There are now thousands of people worldwide who have successfully completed this type of combined program.

Some of you may be wondering if Redux can be used by normal-weight smokers to reduce the possibility of weight gain should they choose to quit. It makes no difference how much people weigh when they quit; everyone has a tendency to gain weight after smoking cessation. In 1995, a study was published in the *American Journal of Clinical Nutrition* discussing this issue. Prozac was also a variable in the study. In the study, 144 normal-weight women were separated into three groups. One group quit smoking while taking Redux, another did so while taking Prozac, and the third (control group) quit smoking while taking a placebo. One month after quitting smoking, the placebo group had gained the most weight. After three months, the Redux group had gained only 1–2 pounds, while the Prozac group had gained 5 pounds and the control group had gained 7 pounds! Three months after the drugs were stopped, weight gain in the Redux and Prozac groups matched that in the control group. This study demonstrates that, although this is not one of its official indications, Redux can actually work for normal-weight individuals who want to stop smoking without gaining weight. It also illustrates the importance of using Redux for the extended period prescribed in my ten-step "Quit and Lose" program.

This plan will work for you if your desire to quit smoking matches your desire to lose weight. It's time now for you to take control of your health. Stop smoking and lose weight!

DID YOU KNOW . . .

- 50% of all smokers die prematurely.
- The temperature in a smoker's mouth can reach up to 120 degrees. So much for smoking being "cool."
- As many women smoke as men.
- Six times fewer African-American teenagers smoke than white teenagers.
- The tobacco companies spend $3 billion a year in advertising.
- Besides lung cancer, smoking causes cancer of the bladder, the mouth and throat, the esophagus, the stomach, and the pancreas.
- Health-care costs for smoking-related illness are $50 billion a year!

Chapter 12

Drugs That Cause Weight Gain

Three pounds gained last week, 21 pounds total—all in the past six weeks! Despite no personal history of obesity and no family history of obesity, you find yourself eating everything in sight—day and night! As a lifelong fitness enthusiast, you see your washboard abdominal muscles fading fast under a blanket of fat. Your shirt buttons are stressed like bridge cables laden with holiday traffic. You seek advice from friends, but their encouraging words can't stop the weight-gain onslaught. Chocolate and cookies replace salad and whole wheat bread. Feelings of "wellness" give way to depression and tears.

The alarm goes off; it's time to wake up. Except this is no dream—it's real. It happened to C.R., a 35-year-old realtor. She went from 145 pounds to 166 pounds in just six short weeks, for no apparent reason. After a great deal of thought, and even more frustration, C.R. began to suspect a recently prescribed medication, amitriptyline. This is a drug that's commonly used to treat depression and chronic pain. I recommended that she speak to her neurologist about stopping amitriptyline, because it has been known to cause weight gain in a fair amount of cases. After checking with her neurologist, she tried another medication. She still didn't lose the excess weight, even when taking phen/fen. In fact, she was now up to 169 pounds.

After three weeks, C.R. came back into my office—all smiles. She had lost seven pounds and was feeling much better. "What happened?" I asked. Enthusiastically, she replied, "I called my pharmacist and he said that the medicine I take to help me sleep, alprazolam, can cause weight gain. I stopped taking the drug." I didn't know that. In fact, when I researched the medication I was surprised to find that not only was alprazolam known to cause weight gain, but it can sometimes cause weight loss! After reflecting on C.R.'s case, I felt the weight gain was probably a result of combining the alprazolam and amitriptyline, which should not have been used together in the first place.

The whole situation was very ironic. Here was a woman who had never been overweight, finding herself gaining weight uncontrollably and becoming increasingly depressed—all because of a medication that was supposed to help her depression! The amitriptyline was the real culprit here, in more ways than one. Not only did the drug act as a catalyst for her weight gain, but it also made it unusually difficult to "bounce back." It even blocked the effects of the phen/fen. C.R. didn't lose the weight when she first stopped taking amitriptyline, because she was depressed. When she switched to fluoxetine, another antidepressant, she was in a better frame of mind to lose the unwanted pounds. This demonstrates how depression and weight gain are intertwined.

There are many medications that can cause weight gain. If you feel that a medication you are taking may be causing you to gain weight or preventing you from losing weight, talk to your doctor or pharmacist. *You cannot lose weight and gain weight at the same time!* Taking Redux simultaneously with amitriptyline, for instance, is not recommended, because you will not lose weight. The amitriptyline will dominate.

Drugs can cause weight gain by any one of these mechanisms:

- By increasing appetite by stimulating the appetite center of the hypothalamus
- By increasing the amount of extra-cellular water in the body, also known as edema
- Indirectly, by stimulating a hormone that causes weight gain
- By unknown mechanisms

Most medications that cause weight gain fall into the last category. We simply do not know why they cause weight gain!

Let's take a closer look at the most common drugs in each of these four categories. A list of some other drugs that cause weight gain, in lesser numbers, will follow. Keep in mind that some of these drugs can be classified in more than one category. In most cases, the brand names are used throughout. Check with your pharmacist to find the correct chemical name for any medications you may be taking.

DRUGS THAT INCREASE APPETITE

Corticosteroids. Commonly called just "steroids," these are used to treat such illnesses as certain cancers and inflammatory illnesses, among others. These are not to be confused with the anabolic steroids abused by athletes. (Incidentally, anabolic steroids also cause weight gain.) Corticosteroids cause a particular type of obesity called "cushinoid." This type of obesity is often characterized by special clinical features, including enlarged cheeks and a fat pad on the back. Unfortunately, these are drugs that treat serious illnesses. *Under no circumstances should these drugs be stopped without consulting your doctor, even if you are gaining weight.* Short-term use of steroids usually does not cause weight gain, except for slight fluid retention.

Estrogens. These female hormones can cause weight gain, but they are also implicated in weight loss. Sometimes it's the progesterone in some birth-control and estrogen-replacement pills that causes water to be retained. This is a large topic that should be addressed with your gynecologist. One thing is very clear: For many postmenopausal women, weight gain is natural. Sometimes the extra body weight is worsened by estrogen-replacement pills. The same holds true for many premenopausal women starting birth-control pills; they often gain weight as well. Many fertility drugs also have been known to cause weight gain. It is crucial that you work with a gynecologist who understands your weight-loss needs. M.J., a 32-year-old woman undergoing infertility treatment, gained 15 pounds on clomiphene. She said the drug made her ovaries feel like bowling balls. The type of medication and dose must be tailored individually. Again, do not stop medication abruptly yourself.

Antidepressants. Any antidepressant drug can cause weight gain. However, in some cases, as with Prozac, the medicine may work similarly to Redux and cause weight loss. The antidepressants to be most concerned with, in terms of weight gain, are the tricyclic antidepressants. These include amitriptyline (the drug C.R. was taking), imipramine, and doxepin, just to name a few. We already know that people in a depressed state of mind have a more difficult time losing weight. Unfortunately, being on a tricyclic antidepressant can preclude weight loss. A new antidepressant that is not a tricyclic and has been found to cause weight gain in only one in 50 patients is buproprion.

DRUGS THAT CAUSE WATER RETENTION

Antihypertensives. These blood-pressure medications include certain calcium channel blockers and beta blockers. With water retention, the first clues of weight gain are located in the extremities—your shoes and rings won't fit! Female hormones and steroids also can cause water retention.

DRUGS THAT CAUSE WEIGHT GAIN BY INDIRECT ACTION

Oral hypoglycemic agents. These are drugs used to treat adult-onset diabetes. They stimulate the pancreas to secrete the hormone insulin. As you may recall, insulin is the hormone that triggers hunger. This partially explains why adult-onset diabetics rarely lose weight. There are several recently released medications that may serve these patients better, or at least enable them to cut down on their dosage of these potent "fat depositors."

DRUGS THAT CAUSE WEIGHT GAIN BY UNKNOWN MECHANISMS

Antihistamines. Astemizole (Hismanal), a popular non-sedating antihistamine, can cause weight gain. However, this is uncommon, and the weight gain is usually minimal.

Other drugs implicated in weight gain include methyldopa (Aldomet), clonidine (Catapres), guanadrel sulfate (Hylorel), lithium carbonate (Eskalith), thioridazine (Mellaril), and alprazolam (Xanax).

Again, if you aren't sure whether a medication you are currently taking causes weight gain, check with your doctor or pharmacist. Your pharmacist can usually furnish a computer printout of the side effects of your medication. If you are taking any of the medicines listed above, perhaps a different medication can be prescribed. If not, perhaps the dosage can be adjusted—weight gain can be a "dose-dependent" phenomenon. The more drugs you have in your body, the more likely you will be to experience side effects. Sometimes you can go on a drug holiday, an interim period off the medication. If you can't change the medication, perhaps you should wait until you no longer require the drug before you attempt weight loss. At least you will know why you are having so much difficulty losing weight.

Finally, it is your responsibility to know if the medication you take has the potential to cause weight gain. Remember, you can't drive with one foot pressed on the accelerator and the other pressed on the brake!

DID YOU KNOW . . .

• A major side effect of diabetes medication is hypoglycemia, or low blood sugar.

• Propranolol, a commonly used drug for high blood pressure, can cause depression.

• There are rare tumors of the pancreas, adrenal gland, and brain that can cause obesity.

• Nonsedating antihistamines, such as astemizole (Hismanal), do not enter your brain and therefore don't make you tired the way diphenhydramine (Benadryl) can.

• Birth-control pills can cause stroke, and smoking increases the risk.

Chapter 13

Questions and Answers

One of the wonderful aspects of being in the health care profession is the constant stimulation that patients provide, both emotionally and intellectually. Redux has provided the impetus for establishing a whole new countrywide weight-loss dialogue between patients and physicians. The following questions, which are actual questions posed by my patients, are part of this new trend.

1. *I am currently taking Prozac (fluoxetine), an antidepressant, for depression. I am 50 to 60 pounds overweight and am a candidate for Redux. Can I take the two medications at the same time?*
Both Prozac and Redux work by elevating the level of the neurotransmitter serotonin in the brain. As was noted in Chapter 4 regarding drug interactions, taking Prozac and Redux together can cause a paradoxical reaction, the "serotonin syndrome," during which the serotonin level is so high that

an acute agitated state might ensue. It seems that there is a serotonin threshold that can be breached by combining the two serotonin-elevating drugs. The expected calming effects of Prozac are then expressed in the opposite fashion: agitation. It is necessary for you and your physician to evaluate your individual case; however, I would not use the two drugs at the same time until further research and clinical experience are available.

2. Is it true that I need to drink eight glasses of water a day to clear my body of toxins if I take Redux?
The body regulates perfectly the daily amount of water you need. In fact, drinking too much water can put excess stress on the kidneys. In people who follow starvation diets, body toxins are produced in the form of broken-down muscle proteins caused by the body's using muscle proteins for energy. *The Redux™ Revolution* does not advocate starvation, hence toxins will not develop. Therefore, drink as much water as your body "tells you" to drink.

3. Is Redux addictive?
Unlike amphetamines, Redux doesn't have addicting properties. However, as a precaution, I do not prescribe weight-loss medications to people who have a history of drug and/ or alcohol abuse.

4. I am a police officer subject to random urine tests. Will Redux show up in a urine sample?
Although it is not an amphetamine, Redux has a biochemical structure that is similar to amphetamines, which are banned for use by law enforcement officials. Using a banned substance can result in immediate dismissal. With the usual drug-testing protocol, any positive test result must be confirmed

with a second, more sophisticated test. If you take Redux, and should the initial screen be positive, the confirmatory second test would be negative. Your personal medical doctor, as well as any physicians involved with your police department, should be advised that you are taking Redux before the testing procedure.

5. Is there any weight-loss advantage gained by going on a low-calorie diet while taking Redux?
The *Redux™ Revolution* does not advocate any type of severe calorie restriction. Severe calorie restriction does not hasten weight loss and is unhealthy. Furthermore, recent research suggests that low-calorie diets can damage the heart. In fact, one study has actually shown that Redux does not work well when used in conjunction with a low-calorie diet (under 800 calories).

6. I am not overweight, nor is my wife. We have a six-month-old son. What are his chances of being overweight?
The odds are one in ten that the baby will be overweight. Had you both been overweight, his chances would have been eight in ten!

7. Will Redux interfere with the effectiveness of my birth-control pills?
There is no known interaction between the two medications.

8. I am 35 years old and have been gaining weight for the past two years. I lack energy and my hair has become coarse and is falling out! What should I do?
It sounds like you may be suffering from a condition called hypothyroidism: an underactive thyroid. The thyroid gland is a shieldlike structure located below the Adam's apple at the

front of the neck. Upon receiving a signal from the brain, it releases the hormone thyroxine, which helps control metabolism. When the gland does not work well, which may happen for a variety of medical reasons, less hormone is produced and you become hypothyroid. If you have symptoms of sluggishness and hair changes, and perhaps have noticed that your face is getting puffier, see your doctor for a simple blood test to rule out this condition. Incidentally, any woman who experiences a sudden weight gain should have her thyroid status checked.

9. *How often should I take Redux, and what happens if I miss a dose?*
Redux is taken twice a day. It is most beneficial to adhere to the suggested dose regimen. However, if you miss a dose there are no harmful consequences. You might notice a temporary increase in your appetite, which will diminish when you resume your regular dose of Redux.

10. *I am an adult-onset diabetic. Will Redux have any effect on my blood sugar level? Will it alter the dose requirements of my insulin?*
As we noted in Chapter 10, recent research shows that Redux can have a favorable effect on diabetes. Although the mechanism of this action is unclear, it is known that Redux decreases the liver's ability to release sugar into the bloodstream, hence lowering blood sugar. Of course, weight loss, brought about by Redux, will in and of itself lower blood sugar levels. The decrease in blood sugar levels may lower the dosage of medication required to control your diabetes, but adjustment of dosage should be done only on the advice of your doctor.

11. *Will Redux interact with the antihistamines I take for my allergies?*
In general, there are two types of antihistamines. One type is the sedating antihistamines, which can make you tired. These are an older type of antihistamine and include diphenhydramine (Benadryl) and clemastine (Tavist). Redux should be used with caution when taking these medications because they can affect the brain to induce sleep. Redux, which exerts its influence on the hypothalamus, where a sleep center is located, has lethargy as one of its side effects. Taking the two drugs together can make you more likely to be tired, and you should avoid driving or operating potentially dangerous machinery while on the medications. On the other hand, Redux can probably be used with antihistamines of the other type, which are newer and nonsedating. These include terfenadine (Seldane), astemizole (Hismanal), and loratidine (Claritin). Let your doctor know if you are taking *any* over-the-counter medications before taking Redux.

12. *Can I take Redux with decongestants?*
Yes. But I would not use decongestants if I were taking phentermine. They both have "stimulant" qualities; they may make you jittery and may prevent sleep if taken at the same time.

13. *I am going through menopause. Will Redux work for me?*
Menopause is a time when many women gain weight, for reasons that are largely unknown. Redux works on the appetite center of the brain and is not affected by the hormonal changes of menopause.

14. *I am 60 years old. Am I a candidate for Redux?*
Many of the supporting studies submitted to the FDA for

Redux's approval included case studies of patients in their 70s who were successful in losing weight on Redux. Weight loss is not age-dependent. You can lose weight at any age.

15. *I plan to go on vacation and sit in the sun. Will Redux affect my skin's reaction to sunlight?*
Many drugs can cause photosensitivity, which occurs when the medication itself sensitizes the skin to the ultraviolet rays of the sun. It makes the skin behave like a sun "magnet" and can cause irritating and severe sun rash. Redux is not known to cause photosensitivity reaction in any large numbers of people. However, try to avoid excessive sun exposure, as it ages the skin and causes skin cancers, such as melanoma.

16. *Do I need to have periodic blood tests while on Redux?*
Periodic blood tests are not necessary while taking Redux.

17. *Can I stop taking Redux abruptly?*
No medication should ever be discontinued without consulting with your doctor. Although there is nothing inherently harmful in stopping Redux abruptly, this decision should be made within the patient/doctor relationship.

18. *Does ephedrine cause weight loss?*
Ephedrine is the chief component in Chinese weight-loss herbs and is currently a widely used street drug with definite abuse potential. In a double-blind study published in the *International Journal of Obesity* (1985), it was concluded that ephedrine does not cause weight loss. It is dangerous and has caused deaths from heart attacks. The FDA is looking into changing its over-the-counter status.

19. *I have a friend who many years ago took thyroid hormone for weight loss. What's the difference between thyroid hormone and Redux?*

Thyroid hormone was popular 20 to 30 years ago as a prescription weight-loss medication. It was hoped that taking thyroid hormone would raise the patient's metabolic rate and burn fat. Unfortunately, it did neither and caused loss of muscle instead. Redux, on the other hand, causes weight loss by its actions on the appetite center in the brain and does not cause muscle loss.

20. *I drink five cups of coffee per day. Does caffeine interfere with Redux?*

Caffeine and Redux do not interact with each other, nor does caffeine in the form of coffee, tea, or chocolate interfere with the action of Redux.

21. *I take ginseng and vitamins. Will Redux interfere?*

Redux does not interact with either ginseng or vitamins, and you may take them together.

22. *My friend was given diuretics to lose weight. Can I take her medication?*

No! Diuretics cause only temporary loss of water and have nothing to do with fat loss. Some have dangerous side effects and should be taken only under the supervision of your own medical doctor. Incidentally, any water weight lost will be quickly regained.

23. *Does Redux affect my metabolism?*

Unlike amphetamines or thyroid medications, Redux has no effect on your metabolism.

24. *Will Redux have any effect on my sleep?*
Redux does not usually interfere with sleep, but as a side effect of the medication, Redux's effect on sleep varies. In some cases it can promote sleep, while in others it can cause insomnia. Some people also experience dreams that are more vivid than usual.

25. *Can I take aspirin or Motrin with Redux?*
There have been no reported interactions between Redux and popular pain medications. It is safe to use them together.

26. *Can I have alcoholic beverages while taking Redux?*
Both Redux and alcohol act on the central nervous system. The combination of Redux and alcohol can synergistically increase the severity and frequency of side effects of Redux, including to lethargy, memory loss, and sleep disturbances. Therefore, I do not recommend drinking alcohol while taking Redux.

27. *Can I exceed the recommended dose of Redux in order to lose more weight?*
The manufacturer's established dose of Redux allows for the optimal balance of effectiveness and safety. There is no evidence that more weight loss can be attained by taking a higher dose of Redux. Taking Redux at higher doses is unsafe and is not recommended. Also, be sure never to take Redux with other weight-loss medications!

28. *I have asthma. Can Redux make my asthma worse?*
Redux has no effect on asthma. However, if you take medication for asthma—or for any other condition—make sure that the doctor prescribing the Redux is aware of all the med-

ications you are taking, including over-the-counter medications.

29. *Can I take Redux on an empty stomach, or must I take it with a meal?*
Food has very little effect on the absorption of Redux. It makes no difference whether you take it on a full or empty stomach.

30. *At what age can I start using Redux?*
It is generally thought to be safe for anyone over the age of 18 to take Redux.

31. *Does Redux work for both men and women?*
Redux works equally well in men and women.

32. *Is there a generic form of Redux?*
No. Because Redux is a new medication in this country, a generic equivalent will not be available in the United States for some years.

33. *The phen/fen regimen did not work for me. Am I still a candidate for Redux?*
Although fenfluramine, one-half of the phen/fen regimen, has some chemical similarities to Redux (dexfenfluramine), Redux should be considered a totally different treatment option for obesity. Therefore, you may be a candidate for Redux provided you fit the criteria outlined by the FDA (see Chapter 3).

34. *I know that Redux can cause abdominal discomfort. Does this lead to ulcers?*
No. The use of Redux does not cause ulcers.

Bibliography

Chapter 1: What Is the Redux Revolution?

Atkinson, R.L., and J.S. Hubbard. "Report on the NIH Workshop on Pharmacologic Treatment of Obesity." *American Journal of Clinical Nutrition*, Aug: 60 (1994) 153–156.

Bruch, Hilde, M.D. *Eating Disorders: Obesity, Anorexia Nervosa, and the Person Within.* New York: Basic Books, 1973.

Stunkard, Albert J., M.D. *Obesity.* Philadelphia: W. B. Saunders, 1980.

Chapter 2: Designer Genes

Arslanian, Silva, and Chittiwat Suprasongsin. "Insulin Sensitivity, Lipids, and Body Composition in Childhood: Is

Syndrome X Present?" *Journal of Clinical Endocrinology and Metabolism*, Vol. 81, No. 3, 1058–1062.

Bennett, William Ira, M.D. "Beyond Overeating." *New England Journal of Medicine (NEJM)*, Vol. 332 (1995) 673–674.

Considine, Robert V., Ph.D., et al. "Serum Immunoreactive-Leptin Concentrations in Normal Weight and Obese Humans." *NEJM*, Vol. 334 (1996) 292–295.

Considine, Robert V., Ph.D., and José F. Caro, M.D. "Serum Immunoreactive-Leptin Concentrations in Normal Weight and Obese Humans." (Letter) *NEJM*, Vol. 334 (1996) 1544.

Leibowitz, S.F., et al. "Neurochemical/Neuroendocrine Systems in the Brain Controlling Macronutrient Intake and Metabolism." *Trends in Neuroscience*, Vol. 15 (1992) 491–497.

Lewis, D.E., et al. "Intense Exercise and Food Restriction Cause Similar Hypothalamic Neuropeptide Y Increases in Rats." *American Journal of Physiology*, Vol. 264 (1993) 279–284.

Pijl, Hanno, M.D., Ph.D., et al. "Serum Immunoreactive-Leptin Concentrations in Normal Weight and Obese Humans." (Letter) *NEJM*, Vol. 334 (1996) 1544.

Reaven, G.M. "Insulin Resistance Hyperinsulinemia, Hypertriglyceridemia, and Hypertension: Parallels Between Human Disease and Rodent Models." *Diabetes Care,* Vol. 14 (1991) 195–202.

Reaven, G.M. "Role of Insulin Resistance in Human Disease." *Diabetes,* Vol. 37 (1988) 1595–1607.

Rohner-Jeanrenaud, F., and B. Jeanrenaud. "Obesity, Leptin, and the Brain." *NEJM*, Vol. 334 (1996) 324–325.

Stewart, Murray W., et al. "Syndrome X in First Degree Relatives of NIDDM Patients." *Diabetes Care*, Vol. 18 (1995) 1020–1022.

Zhang, Y., et al. "Positional Cloning of the Mouse Obese Gene and Its Human Homologue." *Nature*, Vol. 372 (1994) 425–432.

Chapter 3: Redux to the Rescue

Bremer, J., et al. "Dexfenfluramine (Redux) Reduces Cardiovascular Risk Factors." *International Journal of Obesity and Related Metabolic Disorders*, Vol. 18 (1994) 199–205.

Brindley, D.N., and J.C. Russel. "Metabolic Abnormalities Linked to Obesity: Effects of Dexfenfluramine in the Corpulent Rat." *Metabolism*, Vol. 44 (1995) 23–27.

Guy-Grand, Bernard, et al. "International Trial of Long-Term Dexfenfluramine in Obesity." *The Lancet*, Nov. 11, 1989, 1142–1145.

Holdaway, I., et al. "Effect of Dexfenfluramine on Body Weight, Blood Pressure, Insulin Resistance, and Serum Cholesterol in Obese Individuals." *International Journal of Obesity and Related Metabolic Disorders*, Vol. 19 (1995) 739–741.

McCann, Una, et al. "Dexfenfluramine and Serotonin Neurotoxicity: Further Preclinical Evidence That Clinical Caution Is Indicated." *Journal of Pharmacology and Experimental Therapeutics*, Vol. 269 (2) (May 1994) 792–798.

Noach, E.L. "Appetite Regulation by Serotonergic Mechanisms and the Effects of Dexfenfluramine." *NEJM*, Vol. 45 (1994) 123–133.

O'Connor, H.T., et al. "Dexfenfluramine Treatment of Obesity: A Double-Blind Trial with Posttrial Follow-up." *International Journal of Obesity and Related Metabolic Disorders*, Vol. 19 (1995) 181–189.

Recasens, M.A., et al. "Effect of Dexfenfluramine on Energy Expenditure in Obese Patients on a Very Low Calorie

Diet." *International Journal of Obesity and Related Metabolic Disorders*, Vol. 19 (1995) 162–168.

Stahl, K.A., and T.F. Imperiale. "An Overview of the Efficiency and Safety of Fenfluramine and Mazindol in the Treatment of Obesity." *Archives of Family Medicine*, Vol. 2 (1993) 1033–1038.

Stewart, G.O., et al. "Dexfenfluramine (Redux) in Type II Diabetes: Effect on Weight and Diabetes Control." *Medical Journal of Australia*, Vol. 158 (1993) 167–169.

Stunkard, Albert J., M.D. *Obesity*. Philadelphia: W. B. Saunders, 1980.

Van Itallie, T.B. "The Role of Dexfenfluramine in the Regulation of Energy Balance. Introduction." *Metabolism*, Vol. 44 (1995) 1–3.

Voelker, R. "Ambulatory Android Overweight Population with an Overconsumption of Snacks." *International Journal of Obesity and Related Metabolic Disorders*, Vol. 19 (May 1995) 299–304.

Chapter 4: Redux: Safety, Side Effects, and Risks

Cacoub, P., et al. "Pulmonary Hypertension and Dexfenfluramine." *European Journal of Clinical Pharmacology*, Vol. 48 (1995) 81–83.

Herve, P., et al. "Increased Plasma Serotonin in Primary Pulmonary Hypertension." *American Journal of Medicine*, Vol. 99 (1995) 249–254.

Lasagna, Louis. "Drugs in the Treatment of Obesity," in Albert J. Stunkard, M.D., *Obesity*. Philadelphia: W. B. Saunders, 1980.

Naeije, R., et al. "Effects of Dexfenfluramine on Hypoxic Pulmonary Vasoconstriction and Embolic Pulmonary Hypertension in Dogs." *American Journal of Respiratory Critical Care Medicine*, Vol. 151 (1995) 692–697.

Physicians' Desk Reference. 50th ed. Montvale, N.J.: Medical Economics Data Production Company, 1996.

Ricaurte, George, et al. "Dexfenfluramine Neurotoxicity in the Brains of Nonhuman Primates." *The Lancet*, Vol. 338 (1991) 1487–1488.

Sandage, B., Jr., et al. "Review of Dexfenfluramine Efficacy and Safety." Interneuron Pharmaceuticals, Inc., Lexington, Mass. 02173, U.S.A., and Servier Laboratories, Paris BP126, France.

Thomas, S.H., et al. "Appetite Suppressants and Primary Pulmonary Hypertension in the United Kingdom." *British Heart Journal*, Vol. 74 (1995) 660–663.

Tournuliet, A.C., et al. "Major Depression During Dexfenfluramine Treatment." *International Journal of Obesity and Related Metabolic Disorders*, Vol. 18 (1994) 650.

Chapter 5: Redux and Your Diet

Considine, Robert V., et al. "Serum Immunoreactive-Leptin Concentrations in Normal Weight and Obese Humans." *NEJM*, Vol. 334 (1996) 292–295.

Cugini, P., et al. "Chronobiometric Identification of Disorders of Hunger Sensation in Essential Obesity: Therapeutic Effects of Dexfenfluramine." *Metabolism*, Vol. 44 (1995) 50–56.

Lafreniere, F., et al. "Effects of Dexfenfluramine Treatment on Body Weight and Postprandial Thermogenesis in Obese Subjects: A Double-Blind Placebo-Controlled Study. *International Journal of Obesity and Related Metabolic Disorders*, Vol. 17 (1993) 25–30.

Mathus-Vliegen, L.M., and A.M. Res. "Dexfenfluramine Influences Dietary Compliance and Eating Behavior, but Dietary Instruction May Overrule Its Effect on Food Selection in Obese Subjects." *Journal of the American Dietary Association*, Vol. 93 (1993) 1163–1165.

Recasens, M.A., et al. "Effect of Dexfenfluramine on Energy Expenditure in Obese Patients on a Very Low Calorie Diet." *International Journal of Obesity and Related Metabolic Disorders*, Vol. 19 (1995) 162–168.

Scalfi, L., et al. "The Acute Effect of Dexfenfluramine on Resting Metabolic Rate and Postprandial Thermogenesis in Obese Subjects: A Double-Blind Placebo-Controlled Study." *International Journal of Obesity and Related Metabolic Disorders*, Vol. 17 (1993) 91–96.

Stunkard, Albert J., M.D. *Obesity*. Philadelphia: W. B. Saunders, 1980.

Vasquez, J.A., and S.A. Adibi. "Protein Sparing During Treatment of Obesity: Ketogenic Versus Nonketogenic Very Low Calorie Diet." *Metabolism: Clinical and Experimental*, Vol. 41 (1992) 406–414.

Chapter 6: Redux in Motion

Calles-Escandon, J., and E.S. Horton. "The Thermogenic Role of Exercise in the Treatment of Morbid Obesity: A Critical Evaluation." *American Journal of Clinical Nutrition*, Vol. 55 (1992) 533s–537s.

Garrow, J.S. "Exercise in the Treatment of Obesity: A Marginal Contribution." *International Journal of Obesity and Related Metabolic Disorders*, Vol. 19 (1995) 126–129.

Haskell, L. "Exercise and Health," in *Cecil's Textbook of Medicine*. Philadelphia: W. B. Saunders, 1985.

Katzel, Leslie I., et al. "Effects of Weight Loss Versus Aerobic Exercise Training on Risk Factors for Cardiovascular Disease in Healthy, Obese, Middle-aged, and Older Men." *Journal of the American Medical Association*, Vol. 274 (1995) 1915–1921.

King, N.A., and J.E. Blundell. "High-Fat Foods Overcome the Energy Expenditure Induced by High-Intensity Cycling or Running." *European Journal of Clinical Nutrition*, Vol. 49 (1995) 114–123.

Melby, C., et al. "Effect of Acute Resistance Exercise on Postexercise Energy Expenditure and Raising Metabolic Rate." *Journal of Applied Psychology*, Vol. 75 (1993) 1847–1853.

Oletsky, Jerrold M. "Obesity," in *Harrison's Textbook of Medicine*, 9th ed. New York: McGraw Hill, 1980.

Richard, D. "Exercise and the Neurobiological Control of Food Intake and Energy Expenditure." *International Journal of Obesity and Related Metabolic Disorders*, Vol. 19 (1995) 73–79.

Stunkard, Albert J., M.D. *Obesity*. Philadelphia: W. B. Saunders, 1980.

Valtuena, S., et al. "Changes in the Body Composition and Resting Energy Expenditure After Rapid Weight Loss: Is There an Energy-Metabolism Adaption in These Patients?" *International Journal of Obesity and Related Metabolic Disorders*, 19 (1995) 119–125.

Chapter 7: Life After Redux

Atkinson, R.L., and V.S. Hubbard. "Report on the NIH Workshop on Pharmacological Treatment of Obesity." *American Journal of Clinical Nutrition*, Vol. 60 (1994) 153–156.

Kogon, M.M., et al. "Psychological and Metabolic Effects of Dietary Carbohydrates and Dexfenfluramine During a

Low-Energy Diet in Obese Women." *Metabolism*, Vol. 43 (1994) 969–973.

Mathus-Vliegen, L.M. "Dexfenfluramine Influences Dietary and Eating Behaviors of Obese Subjects." *Nutrition Reviews*, Vol. 52, No. 2 (1994) 55–68.

O'Connor, H.T., et al. "Dexfenfluramine Treatment of Obesity: A Double-Blind Trial with Posttrial Follow-up." *International Journal of Obesity and Related Metabolic Disorders*, Vol. 19 (1995) 181–189.

Pfohl, M., et al. "Long-Term Changes of Weight and Cardiovascular Risk Factors After Weight Reduction and Group Therapy with Dexfenfluramine." *International Journal of Obesity and Related Metabolic Disorders*, Vol. 18 (1994) 391–395.

Roberts, S.B. "Abnormalities of Energy Expenditure and the Development of Obesity." *Obesity Research*, suppl. 2 (1995) 155s–163s.

Chapter 8: The Phen/Fen Option

Khan, M., et al. "Successful Appetite Suppression with Fenfluramine in the Obese Diabetic Transplant Patient." *Transplant Process*, Vol. 27 (1995) 975–976.

Physicians' Desk Reference. 50th ed. Montvale, N.J.: Medical Economics Data Production Company, 1996.

Shaw, W.N. "Long-term Treatment of Obese Zucker Rats with LY255582 and Other Appetite Suppressants." *Pharmacological Biochemical Behavior*, Vol. 46 (1993) 653–659.

Stahl, K.A., and T.F. Imperiale. "An Overview of the Efficiency and Safety of Fenfluramine and Mazindol in the Treatment of Obesity." *Archives of Family Medicine*, Vol. 2 (1993) 1033–1038.

Tuominen, S., et al. "Double-Blind Trial Comparing Fen-fluramine, Phentermine and Dietary Advice on Treatment of Obesity." *International Journal of Obesity and Related Metabolic Disorders,* Vol. 14 (1990) 138.

Weintraub, M., et al. "Long-Term Weight Control Study." *Clinical Pharmacology and Therapeutics,* Vol. 51 (1992) 586–646.

Chapter 9: Redux, Your Doctor, and You: Therapeutic Partners

Bruch, Hilde, M.D. *Eating Disorders: Obesity, Anorexia Nervosa, and the Person Within.* New York: Basic Books, 1973.

Hensrud, D.D., et al. "Relationship of Co-morbidities of Obesity to Weight Loss and Four-Year Weight Maintenance/Rebound." *Obesity Research,* suppl. 2 (1995) 217s–222s.

Jeffery, R.W. "Community Programs for Obesity Prevention: The Minnesota Heart Health Program." *Obesity Research,* suppl. 2 (1995) 283s–288s.

Manning, R.M., et al. "The Comparison of Four Weight Reduction Strategies Aimed at Overweight Diabetic Patients." *Diabetic Medicine,* Vol. 12 (1995) 409–415.

Wing, R.R. "Changing Diet and Exercise Behaviors in Individuals at Risk for Weight Gain." *Obesity Research,* suppl. 2 (1995) 277s–282s.

Wurtman, J.J. "Depression and Weight Gain: The Serotonin Connection." *Journal of Affective Disorders,* Vol. 29 (1993) 183–192.

Zung, William K., M.D., et al. "Prevalence of Repressive Symptoms in Primary Care." *Journal of Family Practice,* Vol. 37 (1993) 337–344.

Bibliography

Chapter 10: Health 2000: Saved by the Millennium?

Andersen, P.H., et al. "Influence of Short-term Dexfenfluramine Therapy on Glucose and Lipid Metabolism in Obese Non-diabetic Patients." *Acta Endocrinology,* Vol. 128 (1993) 251–258.

Boardley, D.J., et al. "The Relationship Between Diet, Activity, and Other Factors, and Postpartum Weight Change by Race." *Obstetrics and Gynecology,* Vol. 86 (1995) 834–838.

Freidman, J.E., et al. "Glucose Metabolism in Incubated Human Muscle: Effect of Obesity and Non-Insulin-Dependent Diabetes Mellitus." *Metabolism: Clinical and Experimental,* Vol. 43 (1994) 1047–1054.

Fox, A.A., et al. "Effects of Diet and Exercise on Common Cardiovascular Disease Risk Factors in Moderately Obese Older Women." *American Journal of Clinical Nutrition,* Vol. 63 (1996) 225–233.

Henry, R.R., and S. Genuth. "Forum One: Current Recommendations About Intensification of Metabolic Control in Non-Insulin-Dependent Diabetes Mellitus." *Annals of Internal Medicine,* Vol. 124 (1996) 175–177.

Holdaway, I.M., et al. "Effect of Dexfenfluramine on Body Weight, Blood Pressure, Insulin Resistance and Serum Cholesterol in Obese Individuals." *International Journal of Obesity and Related Metabolic Disorders,* Vol. 19 (1995) 749–751.

Kolanowski, Dr. J., et al. "Effect of Dexfenfluramine Treatment on Body Weight, Blood Pressure, and Noradrenergic Activity in Obese Hypertensive Patients." *European Journal of Clinical Pharmacology,* Vol. 42 (1992) 599–605.

Krentz, A.J., et al. "Basal Intermediary Metabolism in Im-

220

paired Glucose Tolerance and Morbid Obesity." *Diabetes Research*, Vol. 20 (1992) 51–60.

Manson, JoAnn E., et al. "Body Weight and Mortality Among Women." *NEJM*, Vol. 333, No. 11 (September 14, 1995) 677–685.

Richter, W.O., et al. "Dexfenfluramine Inhibits Catechola-mine-Stimulated in Vitro Liposis in Human Fat Cells." *International Journal of Obesity and Related Metabolic Disorders*, Vol.19 (1995) 503–505.

Shaw, G.M., et al. "Risk of Neural Tube Defect–Affected Pregnancy Among Obese Women." *Journal of the American Medical Association*, Vol. 275 (1996) 1093–1096.

Stewart, G.O., et al. "Dexfenfluramine in Type II Diabetes: Effect on Weight and Diabetes Control." *Medical Journal of Australia*, Vol. 158 (1993) 167–169.

U.S. Department of Health and Human Services, Public Health Service. *Healthy People 2000: National Health Promotion and Disease Prevention Objectives*. Boston: Jones & Bartlett Publishers, 1991.

Van Gaal, L.F., et al. "Effects of Dexfenfluramine on Resting Metabolic Rate and Thermogenesis in Premenopausal Obese Women During Therapeutic Weight Reduction." *Metabolism*, Vol. 44 (1995) 42–45.

Werler, M.M., et al. "Pre-Pregnancy Weight in Relation to Risk of Neural Tube Defects." *Journal of the American Medical Association*, Vol. 275 (1996) 1089–1092.

Chapter 11: Redux and Smoking: Quit Now and Lose Weight!

Bjorntorp, P. "Neuroendocrine Abnormalities in Human Obesity." *Metabolism*, Vol. 44 (1995) 38–41.

Califano, J.A., Jr. "The Wrong Way to Stay Slim." *NEJM,* Vol. 333 (1995) 1214–1216.

Flegal, K.M., et al. "The Influence of Smoking Cessation on the Prevalence of Overweight in the United States." *NEJM,* Vol. 333 (1995) 1165–1170.

Gross, J., et al. "Nicotine Replacement: Effects of Post-cessation Weight Gain." *Journal of Consultations in Clinical Psychology,* Vol. 57 (1989) 87–92.

Henningfield, J.E. "Nicotine Medications for Smoking Cessation." *NEJM,* Vol. 333 (1995) 1196–1203.

Rothman, R.B. "Smoking Cessation in a Patient Being Treated with Fenfluramine Plus Phentermine for Simple Obesity." *Journal of Clinical Psychiatry,* Vol. 57 (1996) 92–93.

Spring, B., et al. "Efficacies of Dexfenfluramine and Fluoxetine in Preventing Weight Gain After Smoking Cessation." *American Journal of Clinical Nutrition,* Vol. 62 (1995) 1181-1187.

Chapter 12: Drugs That Cause Weight Gain

Physicians' Desk Reference, 50th ed. Montvale, N.J.: Medical Economics Data Production Company, 1996.

Chapter 13: Questions and Answers

Pasquali, R., et al. "A Controlled Trial Using Ephedrine in the Treatment of Obesity." *International Journal of Obesity,* (1985) 9:93–98.